C000067700

WITCH'S BREW
Secrets of Scents

Other books by Morwyn:

Secrets of a Witch's Coven

Web of Light: Rites for Witches in the New Age

*Green Magic: The Healing Power of Herbs, Talismans, &
Stones*

WITCH'S BREW
Secrets of Scents

MORWYN

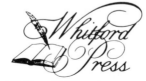

A Division of Schiffer Publishing, Ltd.
77 Lower Valley Road, Atglen, Pennsylvania 19310 USA

*To Ellen, my best friend, for all her
encouragement over the last
twenty-five years.*

Witch's Brew: Secrets of Scents
Copyright © 1995 by Morwyn
Cover Design © by Schiffer Publishing, Ltd.

All rights reserved. No part of this book may be reproduced or used in any form or by any means—graphic, electronic, or mechanical, including photocopying, mimeographing, recording, taping, or information and retrieval systems—without written permission from the publisher.

International Standard Book Number: 0-924608-19-6
Library of Congress Catalog Card Number: 95-68972

Cover Illustration by Steve Ferguson, Colorado Springs, CO

Published by Whitford Press
A Division of Schiffer Publishing, Ltd.
77 Lower Valley Road
Atglen, PA 19310
Manufactured in the United States of America
This book may be purchased from the publisher.
Please include $2.95 postage.
Try your bookstore first.
We are interested in hearing from authors with book ideas
on related subjects.

Contents

Chapter 1:

The Secrets of Scents
The Pervasive Power of Perfume

Pick your favorite time of year. Maybe it is the Fall. What memories does autumn conjure up for you? Perhaps the earthy odor of falling leaves when you crush them underfoot on a walk during a late season rain. Or the smell of smoke curling up into the crisp air from chimneys as the first fires of the season are lighted. The spicy scented apples maturing on the trees, attracting swarms of yellow jackets. Warm and fragrant grapes turning purple in the fields. Mouth-watering kitchen aromas of hot mulled cider steeped with cinnamon and mace, pumpkin pie, and roasting turkey.

Choose another pleasant memory, and recall the image of your mate, significant other, or any person with whom you were ever deeply in love. One of the first things about this person you may remember is the smell of his aftershave, her perfume or hair mousse, and also a barely definable, somewhat musky odor in the other person that somehow drives you wild with desire.

Now change tack and recall a disagreeable or frightening event. Like the time you almost ran into the back of another car on the highway, and how at the last minute you skidded to a halt on the shoulder -- the acrid odor of burning rubber assailing your nostrils.

Or the time you were called into the principal's office for slugging it out with the school bully on the playground. Sidling down the hall to the dreaded seat of authority you still recall the smell of the classrooms and hallways -- freshly sharpened pencils, powdery chalk, school books, gym shoes, half-eaten peanut butter sandwiches mouldering away in lockers, and the peculiar odor of the chemicals the janitors sprinkle on the floor when a child gets sick in the bathroom.

Our memories, indeed, our life experiences are intimately linked to our olfactory sense. Animals particularly have a keen sense of smell. For example, hunting dogs can track their quarry with as little as one billionth of a gram of scent to rely on. In the virtually uninhabited regions of the earth around the Arctic Circle, wildlife will remain about a 20 minute walk away from human intruders because it is only at that distance that they cease to smell us.

Compared to animals, humans are lightweight sniffers. Over thousands of years of evolution we have lost our need to hunt prey with our noses and mark our territories with scent. In contemporary times, we have learned to suppress our odor detecting abilities to protect us from the constant bombardment of competing scents like deodorants, household products, permed hair, synthetic and designer perfumes, not to mention environmental pollutants like smog, insecticides, and other chemical hazards of contemporary life.

Yet our ability to perceive odors still remains one of our most acute senses. For example, newborn babies are able to distinguish the scent of their own mothers' milk after only two days. About ninety-eight per cent of what we smell never reaches our conscious minds, but travels directly through the limbic system, the most primitive part of the brain, to our subconscious minds where odors profoundly affect our emotions. This is why people react strongly, and often irrationally to smells.

In the vignettes presented above, one person may dislike the smells of the schoolroom, while to someone else, the same odors conjure up thoughts of the joy of learning. Whereas I love the fragrances of autumn, these same scents may remind you sadly of a shattered relationship or of a relative who passed away at that time of year.

In the description of the lover, the indefinable musky smell is probably the partner's pheromones, the individual's sexual scent that signals intraspecial attraction and communication. Have you ever met a potential lover for the first time and decided in about thirty seconds whether you were interested in pursuing the relationship? Probably you sensed the other person's pheromones, and on the basis of compatibility decided either to accept or reject the candidate.

Precisely because odors affect our subconscious minds, Witches seek to learn the effects of fragrances and use them to help understand themselves and create changes in their consciousnesses in accordance with their wills. In short, Witches use fragrances to work Magic.

Perfume History

Witches are not the first or only ones to have conceived of using scents to enrich their lives. People always have associated pleasant odors with holy things. For example, Alexander the Great was said to emit a heavenly scent that impregnated all he touched. In the Bible, Paul links sweet smells with those who follow Christ's teachings. Similarly, several great saints were reputed to exude pleasant odors from their bodies and linens. These fragrant emanations were known as "the odor of sanctity."

It is no wonder that as early as 2,000 - 3,000 B.C. ancient civilizations discovered the art of perfumery. Prior to that time, tribes burned fragrant wood at animal and human sacrifices both to mask the stench of roasting flesh and to honor their gods with sweet smoke. Fragrance was considered a mediator between humans and their gods because it proceeded from matter, but was manifested as spirit. In this way, a connection was drawn between humans and gods, and the individual's experiences communicating with the gods was enhanced.

Perfume oils became key ingredients in rituals of baptism and death, and the crowning of kings. In Egypt, dried perfumes were placed with mummies in their tombs in the belief that if the tomb were desecrated and the parts of the body scattered, it could be reassembled on the basis of the accompanying fragrance.

When civilizations discovered that they did not always have to burn woods, resins and other materials to create fragrances but could extract the aromatic essence from substances with oil or water, the perfume industry was born. Perfumiers distilled essences from flowers, fruits, woods, bark, resins and leaves so that people could inhale, ingest, and externally apply the concoctions to their bodies.

They ingested essences for medicinal reasons and sprinkled them in bath water to increase their appeal. For pure pleasure Egyptians added fragrant oils to potpourris and sachets and placed them in containers in which they floated candlewicks. Women even scented their makeup.

Perfumery customs, just like with any other fashion trend, change from culture to culture as well as over time. Ancient Egyptians liked to welcome dinner guests to their homes by handing them fragrant wax cones to place on their heads. In the presence of body heat, the cones slowly melted, covering the honored guests with oozing sweetness.

Egyptians and other ancient peoples, like the Sumerians and Greeks, preferred strong, spicy odors which they extracted in fatty oils. Given the facts that refrigeration did not exist in those times and that oils went rancid quickly, genuine Egyptian blends leaned decidedly on the heavy side for contemporary tastes. This is something you should bear in mind when ordering so-called Egyptian recipes that claim to be replicas of ancient formulas. They would have to be very loosely connected to the original Egyptian formulas in order to be palatable to us.

We usually think of the ancient Hebrews as a strict culture with little time or patience for frills. Yet they traded in aromatics and used them to honor their god. One of the oldest existing fragrance recipes is given in the Bible.[1] It combines spices and exotic scents like stacte and onycha, as well as the more familiar galbanum and frankincense.

Perfumery was practiced as an art throughout the Middle and Far East in ancient times. The Chinese and Japanese designed special scenting racks for hanging their robes prior to participating in religious celebrations. The Japanese were fond of wearing a different fragrance for each day of the week much in the same way that some contemporary Qabalistic Magicians anoint themselves daily with planetary oils. And long before Pledge furniture polish was invented, the Chinese rubbed lemon balm into their furniture wax to produce a fresh, citrusy fragrance.

The Arab physician Avicenna (980-1037) discovered how to use alcohol to distill fragrances from various substances, and revolutionized the art of perfumery. No more extraction in rancid oils! Along with other research into the medicinal values of plants, the Arabs took the theories of the influence of perfume one step further and began to experiment with the effects of essences on human health.

Greek culture picked up where the Egyptians left off. In ancient Greece, men scented themselves even more lavishly than women. When they arrived home from work their wives offered them fragrant baths and body oils and even scented their food and wine. The Greeks loved to splash a different perfume on each part of the body -- one at the throat, another at the temples, yet another between the breasts, under the arms, at the ankles, and on the soles of the feet. They believed that flowers were made from the bodies and blood of their gods and goddesses, and being of such material, could cleanse the body of disease and even rid cities of plague. So they planted their town plazas with flowers and crowned their kings, statues, and even themselves at social functions with wreaths.

Great copiers of culture that they were, the Romans continued and refined Greek fragrance traditions. Crowns of specially chosen leaves and flowers were worn by VIPs on civic occasions, and a citizen could be punished severely for wearing the wrong crown at the wrong time. For example, only a general could sport a wreath of wildflowers and sweet grasses, and only if he had just succeeded in forcing an enemy to raise a siege. On the other hand, myrtle haloes were worn by less instrumental military leaders.

Needless to say, the Romans copiously splashed about fragrances in their baths and at social occasions. Emperor Nero had the dining room of his palace outfitted with spouts cleverly hidden in the ceiling rather like fire prevention water sprinklers in contemporary apartment buildings. When his guests were comfortably wining and dining he would give the order to open the faucets and deluge the revellers with rosewater. Sometimes a flock of doves were released into the room high above the guests' heads, batting their scented wings, and dispersing fragrance into the air.

The Romans may have suffered from something of a "keeping up with the Joneses" complex when it came to scents, especially roses. They used to cover their floors at dinner parties, weddings, and other special occasions with rose petals so that stepping on them released a delightful aroma. In an attempt to outdo each other, they spread petals around so liberally that the practice had to be limited because it depleted the region's rose supply.

Unfortunately, the regulation did not prevent one tragedy from occurring. During the decline of Rome, Heliogabalus, a fourteen-year-old monarch, at his coronation in 218 A.D. ordered rose petals to be showered on his guests from the ceiling. So many thousands of petals were piled on them that celebrants suffocated.

When the Dark Ages descended on Western civilization after the fall of Rome, personal use of fragrances was condemned because in the Medieval Christian Church perfume symbolized the evil Pagan empire. However, anointing oils were still used for sacred rites and at coronations, and symbolic flowers appeared in religious paintings and on tombs.

Returning Crusaders kept alive the interest in perfumery with the exotic fragrances that they brought home from the Orient. Monks studied plants and their essences for their medicinal values, which they called "virtues" and built heavenly herb gardens in their monasteries. In 1190, the French, whose style even then was *avant garde*, formed their own perfume industry and began to regulate it by requiring a fixed number of years of training and experience before an apprentice could become a master perfumier.

During the Renaissance, interest in fragrances quickened. Paracelsus (1493-1541), considered the father of chemical pharmacology and homeopathy, discovered that the value of medicinal plants derived from their chemical composition. By extracting plant essences, he could create powerful medicines to cure disease.

This was also the Age of Discovery when Europeans travelled to new and exotic lands and returned laden with examples of heady scents from the New World like hibiscus, copal and vanilla. Spain, Portugal and Italy, gateways to the West, became bustling perfume-making centers because the raw materials first passed through their domain on the way to European destinations. Animal odors, like musk and castoreum, were refined and shipped to France to scent gloves, and Portugal Essence became the rage in Europe.

Given their geographical and cultural closeness to the Moslem World, the Iberian perfumiers relied, in part, on Middle Eastern recipes.

In 1533, Catherine of Medici moved to France accompanied by her perfume specialists, who in turn, brought with them their expertise to the fledgling French perfume industry.

Perfume was popularized in England by way of the Mary Stuart, Scottish-French connection. During Elizabethan times and throughout the seventeenth century and beyond, country house stillrooms were fashionable. In those days most people lived in the countryside away from town centers. Ladies with access to the abundant flowers and herbs grown in British gardens set aside a small room (or even a cupboard, if no extra room was available) in which they distilled essences of lavender, rose, chamomile, rosemary and other floral delights. They sweetened linens, clothing, furniture and rooms with the concoctions, and the entire family partook of the medicinal values of the essences. Doctors were rare birds, especially in the countryside, and folks had to rely on the healing powers of the botanicals around them to cure their ailments. One charming custom took place every year when country wives gathered in each other's homes to sniff and compare the current year's lavender essence with those of previous seasons.

At Court, the Queen revelled in fragrances and even employed a woman to seek out the best and most fragrant blossoms from nearby gardens for the royal recipes. Queen Elizabeth I was fond of strewing herbs on the floor of her bedroom to sweeten the air, and she wore amber-scented gloves. Tiny, jewelled, metal casting bottles of perfume worn like necklaces were stylish at Court. They were called casting vials because ladies sprinkled fragrances in the air as they walked both for the pleasant odor, and because they thought that nice smells warded off plague and other diseases.

During the Plague years, doctors carried canes with the hollow ends filled with camphor or cloves in the conviction that certain scents kept them from contracting diseases. Centuries later, scientists discovered that essence of clove is a strong antibacterial agent.

The eighteenth century saw the appearance of dandy gentlemen who took fastidious care of themselves. They dressed elaborately and drenched their bodies, hair, and clothing in perfume.

With the nineteenth century and the Victorian Age emerged a kindling of interest in keeping clean and in creating fresh herbal and light flowery scents for soaps, perfumes, and cosmetics. Victorian ideas still influence modern Western attitudes toward cleanliness and odors.

Nonetheless, the twentieth century, like previous eras, has made its own unique contribution to the fragrance industry. Due to the refinements of modern chemistry, polished synthetic perfumes have been developed and aggressively marketed. Fragrances fill our lives from scented toilet paper, stationery and candles to the outgassings of carpeting and plastics. Our senses are bombarded by odors, sometimes sophisticated, but often cloying or harsh.

Perhaps because we are so inundated by strong odors in our daily lives, current trends show that people are tiring of cheap, strong, drugstore perfumes. They are beginning to take an interest in environmental preservation, which means that many are returning to a more natural lifestyle that opts for unscented household and personal cosmetic items. They choose natural essences and environmentally correct synthetics to make their personal statements. Besides appreciating their cosmetic qualities, the public is being drawn to the mysterious power of fragrances for their therapeutic values and ability to alter states of consciousness. In short, consumers are becoming more informed and learning to appreciate fragrances for their intrinsic values.

Perfume Witchery

Witches always have valued the occult virtues of fragrances. These characteristics are called "occult" in the sense that they are hidden from, dismissed, or largely ignored by most people. Witches realize that scent is a form of communication that directly enters the subconscious level of the brain, bypassing, and sometimes overriding conscious communication. In the subconscious mind, scent evokes primal emotions and taps into a wellspring of vivid images and associations. Witches attempt to transmit these perceptions to consciousness because they feel that these recognitions often are more direct, clear, and significant than conscious thoughts. As aromatherapists know, fragrance can instill the body's tissues with new vitality. Mentally, scent can clear the head and foster awareness of esoteric knowledge that may improve a person's own life as well as the existence of humankind. Under the right circumstances, fragrance can be so intoxicating that Witches may be convinced they are inhaling the essence of the divinity.

Furthermore, Witches believe they can use the intrinsic qualities of fragrance to help manifest energy forms and forces of their own device. These created forms and forces reverberate into the Cosmos in order to attract or repel specific influences.

Witches anoint talismans, sigils, candles, pomanders, sachets, sacred stones, ritual apparatus, and their own bodies during ceremonies in order to 1) call upon spirits (or energies), 2) induce visions, 3) stimulate the mind, 4) cause dreams, 5) charge weapons, 6) protect from psychic attack, 7) bring luck, love, money, peace, good health, and other desires. Because fragrances compose a key element of magical operations, anyone aspiring to be an effective Witch, Magician, Shaman, or shape-shifter of any sort must master the occult properties of scents; hence the purpose of this book.

The Language of Flowers

At this point, you may be wondering how we arrive at our specific associations for an almost endless variety of scents. Why do roses stand for love, but the evening primrose symbolizes inconstancy? Some of the meanings of fragrances and the plants from which they derive have been gathered into a collection known as "The Language of Flowers." Popularly it is supposed that this slim compendium originated with Madame de la Tour, who published *Le Langage des Fleurs* around 1840. The origins actually are much more ancient.

Before people could read and write and when they were more in touch with their intuitive natures than we are today, they devised a way to communicate with each other through plants. They developed the interpretations according to the shape, size, fragrance, and other physical characteristics of botanicals. In the ancient world, the Chinese and Japanese sent detailed political and love messages to each other with flower bouquets. Even after the advent of literacy in the West, the largely illiterate peasantry continued to communicate through flowers. Symbolic meanings of flowers were incorporated into folklore and mythology, and eventually art and literature.

Madame de la Tour's book is in part based on this information as well as on the research of Lady Mary Wortley Montagu, wife of the British Ambassador to a Turkish Sultan. In the early 1700's she brought back to England a list of Eastern connotations for flowers that she compiled from interviews with her Oriental friends.

Later in the nineteenth century, as a reflection of their tendency to glorify nature, Victorians seized the idea of a symbolic flower language, and with their usual zeal researched and practiced it as an art. Tussie mussies -- small bouquets of flowers enclosed in a doily or tissue -- were frequently exchanged. These tiny bouquets could convey amazingly complex ideas. For example, a day lily meant "coquetry" while a yellow lily meant a "lie." Whether a flower was presented as a bud or in full flower was significant, as well as the predominant color and texture of the mini-bouquet. Where the flowers were worn on the clothing could convey subtle variations of meaning. Witches today incorporate many of these Victorian attributes of flowers in their fragrance crafting.

Another type of categorization called the Doctrine of Signatures also comes into play. In this system that dates back to the Renaissance, it was observed that certain plant parts resembled parts of the human body in form or color, and were presumed to cure corresponding ailments in humans. Yellow plants were thought to remove bile from the system, red plants cured blood diseases. Bladderwort, that looks like tiny human bladders, was considered to have a beneficial influence on this organ. According to the Doctrine of Signatures, everything that exists on Earth, including plants, is linked to a planet in our solar system. The planets, in turn, are supposed to exercise considerable influences on terrestrial life. All kinds of things besides plants are associated with the planets, including colors, angelic forms, letters of the alphabet, astrological signs, mythical beasts, musical tones, and naturally, scents.

Modern day workers of Magic recognize that because people have believed in these associations for centuries, thought forms have been created and built up around the idea of planetary influences which in turn, have caused these influences to become true, even through originally they may or may not have been. The associations, or correspondences, as they are called in Magic, symbolize these forces. For example, because people have considered honeysuckle, rose and benzoin to be linked with Venus, the planet of love and relationships, wearing honeysuckle, rose and benzoin fragrances attracts love. Actually, there is more to this theory than simple belief, as intrinsic qualities also play an important role. Explanations of these theories lie outside the scope of this book, and may be found in the first volume of this series, *Secrets of a Witch's Coven,* Whitford Press, 1988. Suffice it to say that Ceremonial Magicians surround themselves with the correspondences of the planetary influences they wish to draw in order to charge their senses so that they identify more completely with the planet. Fragrance is one of the most powerful correspondences they use to achieve this aim.

Witches also work with fragrances in rituals and spell casting, but often they use scents and the plants from which they are derived in very concrete ways. They decorate the Sabbat punchbowl or celebratory cake with real or candied flowers. They adorn and scent altars and altar cloths. They anoint talismans, ritual tools, conjure balls and themselves with sacred oils, all by way of aligning themselves with the characteristics that these fragrances represent. Ways to select and blend these components is the topic of the next chapter.

Communication Through Scent: Letter Scents

Undoubtedly there have been times when you wanted to communicate strong emotions to someone else through a letter yet felt that mere words could not express your sentiments adequately. Letter scents can give your words the boost they need to achieve your intent.

As you have already learned, scents affect all people on a subliminal level. Some fragrances, no matter how they impress a person consciously, will have specific and predictable effects on the subconscious mind. Racial memory, or the great human unconscious, as described by Jung and others, is one important reason why scents, as well as other magical phenomena, are influential.

Let me give you an example. I enjoy wearing jasmine perfume because of the heady sweetness and underlying tart, zesty aroma. Jasmine is also a powerful sexual attractant. Recently I was in a gem and mineral store, wearing jasmine perfume lightly dabbed behind my ears and at my heart, when two young women entered. They immediately converged on where I was browsing and sniffed the air. One of them said quite loudly to the other,

"There sure are some strange smells in here today."

"Strong, too," the other replied with a snort.

Soon they huffed out the door and headed across the street. I gazed out at the two unhappy, shuffling figures and realized that they were in great need of love in their lives, and were only venting their frustrations and anger. In spite of their obvious attraction to the scent and its subliminal message, they were unable or unwilling to open themselves to the beauty and enchantment of jasmine, which is known as the "king of flowers" and evokes powerful sensuality. These women were not about to entice a page into their lives, let alone a knight or a king.

You may take advantage of these "scent memories" by adding fragrance in the form of sachets to your letters in order to underscore the written word. You can also express hidden meanings that have nothing to do with the words you write. For example, you can pen a polite response to a man or woman who is interested in dating you, and at the same time through the letter's scent gently tell this person to seek another object of the affections elsewhere (recipe to follow).

To create letter scents you need a mortar and pestle, mixing bowl, spoon, measuring spoons, a handful of botanicals and a few drops of some perfumes. Sometimes you may wish to package your product in colorful wrapping paper or cardstock.

Grind the botanicals to a fine powder with the mortar and pestle, and transfer them to the mixing bowl. All the recipes that follow require 1 tablespoon of cornstarch as a carrier for the oils. According to the ingredients required, combine the pulverized botanicals with the cornstarch, add drops of fragrance, and mix well. Cover the mixture with a lid or piece of paper, and stir well twice a day until the cornstarch absorbs all the oil -- usually no more than three days.

When the mixture matures, write the letter, and sprinkle it with the letter scent. After two hours, brush it away from the paper, seal the letter in an envelope, and mail it. If you are careful to save the used fragrance material in an airtight amber-colored bottle, you can reuse it. Be sure to label the bottle, and only use it again for the exact same purpose.

In some cases – get well, happy birthday, thank you, etc. you may wish the recipient to know that you have spiked the letter and will even want to enclose the letter scent as an envelope sachet gift. Cut a small rectangle from wrapping paper or card stock, and fill it with the appropriate letter scent. Fold up the paper to make a little square envelope, and seal it with glue. Add a drop or two of food coloring to add visual interest to the blend. Insert the envelope inside your greeting card. Envelope sachets make ideal drawer and closet fresheners.

Sometimes you will not wish to have the recipient know that you have scented the letter, for example, when you prepare a job application or wish to compel someone to do your bidding. In these cases, you need only brush the letter scent on the paper and quickly remove it before it has time to penetrate the paper. As an analogy, you can consider that these letter scents are transmitted in "homeopathic doses." Just as the weak amounts of active ingredients in homeopathic medicine produce powerful results, so even a minute vestige of scent can assist you in achieving your aims.

Recipes follow that will enable you to create letter scents for love, birthday greetings, happy anniversary, job application, lottery, to attract business, leave-you-alone, remove negative influences, compel someone to do something, forge a telepathic link, and convey gratitude.

Love

Let's say you just met a wonderful guy and have been out with him once or twice. His birthday is coming up, so you would like to send him a card that at face value is sweet, but not intimate. Subliminally, you wish to let him know that you would very much like to deepen the relationship.

Scent the card with 1 tablespoon cornstarch, a pinch of cassia powder, 3 drops almond oil, 6 drops primrose oil, and 2 drops clover oil.

Time passes, Christmas is around the corner, and the relationship is deepening, yet has not yet become intimate. Scent his holiday greeting card with 1 tablespoon cornstarch, 1/4 teaspoon powdered mistletoe leaves, 1/4 teaspoon ginger powder, 6 drops ambergris oil, 4 drops blue lilac oil, and 4 drops musk oil.

Bingo, you've got him, but you want to keep him hooked. Celebrate your six-month anniversary with a card scented with 1 tablespoon cornstarch, 1/4 teaspoon powdered linden flowers, 6 drops myrrh oil, and 6 drops rose oil.

Your wedding day is here! To keep your love kindled and your husband faithful, give him a wedding card scented with 1 tablespoon cornstarch, 1/4 teaspoon crushed caraway seeds, 1/4 teaspoon cardamom powder, 6 drops carnation oil, 6 drops gardenia oil, 4 drops honeysuckle oil.

In the unlikely event that passion should wane, scent a humorous, sexy card with the ubiquitous 1 tablespoon cornstarch to which you add 8 drops narcissus oil and 4 drops lotus oil.

And (heaven forbid!) you lose him entirely and want the blighter back, scent the letter you write with 1 tablespoon cornstarch to which you add 1/4 teaspoon dragon's blood powder and 8 drops pineapple oil.

Birthday Greetings
To wish someone a very happy birthday you may want to send a card and enclose a home-made sachet created from colorful wrapping paper or cardstock folded as an envelope (explained above) and filled with 1 teaspoon to 1 tablespoon powdered sachet (depending on the size of the sachet). To give the recipient more options than just simply tucking the sachet in a drawer or behind a chair cushion, punch a hole in one corner of the sachet envelope and thread a bright ribbon through the hole. In this way, the recipient can hang the card in a closet or car.

To 1 tablespoon cornstarch, add 6 drops each of two of the oils on the following list. Then mix in 4 drops of one of the recipient's zodiac oils (see zodiac formulas in Appendix II).

Happy Birthday oils: basil, cherry, marjoram, fir, ginger, heather, heliotrope, honeysuckle, marigold, narcissus, tangerine.

Happy Anniversary
To wish a couple a long, happy, and productive life together, on their anniversary send them a card with an envelope sachet made in the same way as the happy birthday formula. Use a zodiac

oil from the sign of the anniversary date. Anniversary oils include: apple blossom, bay, broom, cinnamon, deer's tongue leaves (1/4 teaspoon powdered leaves), vanilla, pikaki, and orange blossom.

Job Application

You are a man who has completed his education and has been working at starter jobs for two or three years. You feel it's time to move up in the world, and you see a marvelous opportunity advertised in the paper. You polish your resume and write a dynamic cover letter. Although you believe that your sterling qualities and outstanding qualifications cannot help but impress a potential boss, it never hurts to enlist a little extra help, right?

Put together a "hire me" sachet, pass it across the application and cover letter very lightly as described above. Remove all vestiges of the sachet, mail the letter, and prepare yourself for the important interview that surely will soon be offered. To 1 tablespoon cornstarch add 10 drops of the following oils. In parentheses I include some specialized attributes:

allspice, cedar, cherry (education), citronella (eloquence in writing -- maybe this is how I got an editor to pay attention to this book!), coriander (shows the light you've been hiding under a bushel), galangal (conquers difficulties -- use it when you know 800 other people have applied for this post), honeysuckle (business, home economics), jasmine, lotus (confers eloquence), marigold (gets respect), musk (shows your self-assuredness), saffron.

Lottery

Despite your best efforts, your application was not received by the cut-off date. What to do for quick cash? There's always the lottery. Put together a sachet with 8 drops of four of the following ingredients mixed into 1 tablespoon cornstarch. Rub the scent on your hands to inspire you before you go to pick your numbers:

almond, anise, basil, bay, cinnamon, clover, frankincense, grape, hyacinth, jasmine, lilac, marigold, peony, poppy, strawberry. Maybe you'll hit the jackpot and won't need that job after all.

Attract Business

For those of you who are shopkeepers and wish to attract more business, I suggest you send to the folks on your mailing list an invitation to an open house, money-off coupon, etc., scented with a mistletoe and bayberry sachet. Combine 4 drops of each oil. To increase walk-in trade even more, add 6 drops of these oils plus 6 drops of clove oil to 1/4 cup water, and wash the outer doorknob of your store with it. Sprinkle the rest of the scented water on the walk and steps leading up to the store. Do this every business day for a month, and watch the clientele flock to your shop. Every time I work a fair with my business, WildWood Fragrances, I sprinkle this formula in front of the booth. Then I sit back and watch the customers gather around my stall.

Repel Negative Influences

The girl who runs the copy machine where you work has been making eyes at you. She works out at your health club and pesters you there, too. What's worse, she found out it was your birthday and baked you a cherry tart in the form of a heart. She's a nice, if rather dim child who means well, but you are definitely attached to Peggy Sue.

Send her a brief and courteous thank-you note scented with "leave-me-alone" sachet. To 1 tablespoon cornstarch add 1/4 teaspoon powdered cinquefoil leaves, 3 drops patchouly oil, 5 drops myrrh oil, and 2 drops frankincense oil.

Banish Negativity

Things being as they are, you are unable to make a payment on a long outstanding account until next month, ten days after the collection agency has threatened to confiscate your car. What to do? Write them a polite note explaining your predicament and scent it with 1 tablespoon cornstarch, 10 drops patchouly oil, 5 drops geranium oil, and five drops bay oil.

Get Well

From time to time, a relative or dear friend falls ill, and may even be hospitalized. Send this person a cheery get well greeting with an enclosed envelope sachet that will brighten her/his day, and speed psychic and physical healing. Choose 6 drops total of four of the following oils and add to the cornstarch:

apricot (insures a long life), poplar buds (1/4 teaspoon powdered buds), benzoin, bergamot, carnation, chamomile (confers strength in adversity), fennel, lavender (a systemic balancer – either the oil or 1/4 teaspoon powdered buds), orange blossom, thyme.

Compelling

Your high school reunion is coming up, and you'd like to see Jane, your former best friend. After high school, she married and moved to a farm in Nebraska, and although you've corresponded you haven't seen her since she graduated. She has three children now, and is busy with the harvest season and doesn't think she can take the time to attend. Still you know she'd have a great time and forget some of her current preoccupations if only she could slip off to Chicago for a few days. Write her a letter and scent it with 1 tablespoon cornstarch, 1/4 teaspoon powdered calamus root, 1/4 teaspoon powdered vervain leaves, and 7 drops each of narcissus and violet oils.

Forge a Telepathic Link

The "compelling" letter worked, and you renewed your friendship with Jane. During the reunion you both realized that besides sharing a lot in common you seem to understand each other's thoughts intuitively -- almost as if you were the sisters neither of you ever had. You both decided to maintain your friendship on all levels, including the telepathic one, and to this end you include sachets in your correspondences to keep the psychic connection alive.

Choose three of any of the following oils, and add 3 drops of each to the cornstarch: bay, blue sonata, camphor, clary sage, clover, cornflower, fern, mimosa, orchid, poppy, rosemary, sandalwood, wisteria.

Gratitude

Finally, you may have occasion to thank someone for helping you, giving you a gift, or for just being nice. Enclose a cornstarch sachet with 1/4 teaspoon powdered grains of paradise, 6 drops rose oil, 2 drops frankincense oil, 3 drops myrrh oil, and 1 drop lavender oil.

Sometimes you will want your sachet to act fast. Oils of peppermint and thyme are quick activators, and almond oil brings immediate blessings. So if you are in a hurry, add 1 drop of any of these to any of the above sachet blends.

More information on sachets follows in Chapter 5.

Chapter 2:

What's In A Smell?

Before taking advantage of the enticingly subliminal qualities of fragrances in order to work Magic, you should understand something about the components of odors and how to identify them. This doesn't mean you need to have a degree in chemistry, but you must be able to recognize some of the scents commonly used in perfumery and develop a sense of how to blend them.

To increase your familiarity with scents, I suggest you put together a personal fragrance vocabulary. Keep a diary, or set of note cards to jot down your impressions. Never experiment with more than three or four fragrances at a time, or the old sniffer could go into "sensory overload" and fail to relay accurate information.

When defining a scent, first categorize it according to the family of odors to which it belongs. For example, it can smell refreshing, like bayberry, citrusy, like tangerine, woodsy, like hemlock, or flowery like peony. Next, describe the scent's distinguishing odor in more detail by using specific descriptive words, examples of which follow later in this chapter.

When sampling fragrances, be aware that many variables can affect your impressions. No scent is pure and simple due to the complexity and variety of ingredients that compose any odor. Even the same species of jasmine, let's say, will differ according to the kind of soil where it was grown, how much sun and water it received, and when it was harvested. Consider yourself an inconsistent factor as well because your perceptions may change according to your mood, the weather, time of day, time of month, season, your physical condition, age, and location.

Ready to experiment? First choose a fragrance and sniff it out of the bottle. Next, dab a few drops on a cotton ball, a blotting pad cut into strips, or a Q-Tip. I prefer a Q-Tip because I can twist a sticky label to the center of it and write on the identification. Sniff the cotton while it is wet, then wait for it to dry, and smell it again. At each stage in the process you may pick up different ideas. Now apply a couple of drops to your wrist, or to the inside of your elbow, wait for it to dry, and sniff again. The first part of the experiment shows how the pure fragrance strikes you, and the second part reveals how it combines with your body chemistry.

Now label your wrist, and wait to see how long the smell persists, and if it changes quality. Note the results in your diary for future reference.

The first list that follows describes families of odors and gives examples. Some categories overlap; others have subsets. The second list suggests some specific vocabulary. As you continue to work with fragrances, you will add other terms to this list.

I. Fragrance Families

1. flowery - orange blossom
2. stimulating - eucalyptus
    subset: sexually stimulating - jasmine
3. refreshing - lavender
    subset: green - pine
    subset: minty - wintergreen
4. citrusy - bergamot
    subset: fruity - strawberry
5. narcotic/intoxicating - musk (also animal-like)
    subset: oriental - ylang-ylang
6. animal-like - civet
    subset: earthy - chypre
7. herby - thyme
    subset: fernlike - fougere

8. woodsy - sandalwood. Woodsy and green sometimes are combined in the same category.
9. spicy - clove
10. grassy - new mown hay.

II. Perfume Vocabulary

Here are some examples of descriptive words you can use to help characterize scents. Over time, you will add many more terms to this list:

apple-scented, aromatic, balsamic, bitter, cheesy, cool, crisp, dead, deep, distinctive, feety, fetid, fragrant, fresh, fruity, grassy, harsh, heady, heavy, honey-like, hot, icy, intense, leathery, lemony, licorice-like, light, medicinal, milky, minty, musky, piercing, rancid, rank, rich, ripe, sensual, shallow, sharp, snappy, soft, sour, spicy, sweet, violet-like, warm, waxy, no fragrance at all.

Aromatherapists further classify scents according to a yin (feminine) / yang (masculine) scale. No fragrance is exclusively yin or yang, although at the extremes, violet is mostly yin and civet is decidedly yang.

How long an aroma lasts on you is due only in part to your body chemistry. The rest is a question of natural evaporation rates and intensities. For example, civet is intense and evaporates slowly, while lily-of-the-valley and eucalyptus evaporate quickly. However, lily-of-the-valley is not particularly intense, while eucalyptus is moderately so. Experiment and rate your personal findings on a scale of one to ten. Trust your impressions.

Here is my 10-point system for organizing fragrance information on index cards. From my own index cards I copied much of the information for Appendix I of this book.

Fragrance Name

1. Latin name; Common Names.
2. Origin.
3. Brand.
4. Natural or Synthetic.
5. Yin/yang Rating.
6. Evaporation Rate.
7. Intensity Rating.

8. Family Classification.
9. Description.
10. Further Comments.

Notice that on the index card I mark a space for origin. It is possible to use well over 4,000 scented materials in perfumery. Don't let this staggering number daunt you. Even the best noses in the business stick to less than 400. As an amateur, if you develop a palette of around 50, you can congratulate yourself on being well-rounded.

Under "Further Comments" you can compare the fragrance to other similar aromas, give your impressions of how the scent changed for you over time, or note how you might like to use it in a blend. If you feel like researching the fragrance, you can add historical details such as the fact that it was an important ingredient of some famous *eau d'cologne*, or that it combines well with certain other scents, or that it is found only on some obscure island.

It is important to identify the brand you are sampling. I find that many fragrances vary considerably from supplier to supplier. For example, the honeysuckle I purchase from two separate companies is so different that most people cannot recognize them as the same scent.

Whether the fragrance is extracted from organic matter or concocted in a laboratory also makes a difference. These days, you will find marketers are cashing in on the back-to-basics-back-to-nature craze. Companies tout their products as "natural essences" and "pure perfumes." The following list of definitions will help you understand what exactly you are sniffing at and buying.

Essential Oils

These oils form naturally within a plant while it is young, up to the time it blooms. Then the formation of essential oils ceases. Some essential oils must be extracted as soon as the plant is picked, or their properties will change. The properties of other oils vary according to the time of day (or night!) when they are harvested. Still others possess different qualities, depending on the plant part from which they are extracted. In perfumery, essential oils are also known as essences. However, most essences only contain 15% - 30% essential oil. The rest is cut with alcohol.

You can run several tests to see whether a substance is really an essential oil:

1) Put a drop on a piece of paper or cloth. Since essential oils are volatile, the stain should disappear within a few minutes to a few days. If the stain stays around longer, it is probably a synthetic -- in which case, let's hope you didn't use your best white shirt for the experiment!

2) Drop some of the oil in water. It should not dissolve, as oil and water do not mix.

3) Essential oils will dissolve partly in vinegar.

4) They are readily soluble in alcohol.

5) They mix well with vegetable oils.

Synthetics

The chemical components of essential oils can be identified and reproduced in laboratories, often more cheaply than essential oils, and certainly in larger quantities.

Synthetics fall into two categories: those which reproduce smells found in nature, and those which do not. A group of chemicals called aldehydes, are an example of the second category. Many designer perfumes are concocted with a mixture of aldehydes and essential oils.

Customers often tell me that they only buy pure, natural essential oils, and wouldn't think of sprinkling any of those nasty chemicals on their bodies. I understand that the idea of natural fragrance is esthetically pleasing. Some scents, especially the herbal ones, can be difficult to find in any other form. Synthetic aromatherapeutic oils can be dangerous to ingest. Essential oils also possess a certain warmth that in my opinion, is impossible to duplicate.

At the same time, we must remember that all fragrance oils, essential or synthetic, are composed of chemicals, and many synthetics are less expensive to produce than their natural counterparts. This is only one incentive for buying them. Synthetics are always stable; that is, their formulas can always be reproduced exactly. In contrast, essential oils depend on soil and growing conditions, and when and where the plants are harvested. Even a little detail like whether the plant grows on the south or north side of a hill can make a big difference in its scent. Botanical harvests vary from year to year, affecting the quality of the rendered oil in the similar way that grape harvests do in winemaking. Moreover, I have found that the quality of many essential oils deteriorates over time more rapidly than many synthetics. These are just some of the variables that can wreak havoc with your perfume blends, especially if you are striving for consistency.

Finally, many natural animal scents such as civet, musk and castoreum are "harvested" by hunting animals and killing them for their scent-producing glands. This is not an ecologically sound policy. Some would argue that to raise crops over and over again in the same location, whether it be for food or fragrance, depletes the soil. Cutting botanicals, including trees, in the wild for their fragrance also upsets the balance of nature. With synthetics you don't suffer these problems.

As to ritual uses of synthetics versus natural fragrances, Richard and Iona Miller in *Magical and Ritual Use of Perfumes* offer an interesting perspective: "While the natural products might seem more esthetically pleasing, our experience has been that the psychological effects of synthetics serve much the same purpose as their natural counterparts." [2] I have found that the Millers' point of view has borne out for me in my own rituals and spellwork.

So it seems, that for ritual work, which is the focus of use of scents in this book, it does not matter whether you choose a synthetic, essential oil, or combination blend.

Here are some other definitions with which to familiarize yourself before you can begin to blend perfumes.

Absolute - a highly concentrated alcohol-soluble fragrance composed of 20% - 80% concretes.

Aldehyde - a combination of essential oils and synthetics in a purified alcohol base.

Attar - a very fragrant, concentrated essential oil, usually created from flower petals, especially roses. "Otto" is another term used to mean attar.

Cologne - named for the city (Cologne, Germany) where the great Italian perfumier, Paul Feminis, lived and applied his trade during the eighteenth century. Colognes are about 3% essential oils in a 70% alcohol base.

Concrete - a waxy, least refined, densest manufactured perfume product derived exclusively from plant material usually soaked in hexane, that is insoluble in water.

Distillation - a method by which essential oils are extracted from plants by steam and condensation with cold water. It takes an enormous amount of plant material to produce essential oil in this way. For example, 1,000 pounds of jasmine petals renders 1 pound of oil.

Enfleurage - a method by which essential oils are extracted from flowers without having to apply high temperatures. The blossoms are soaked in fat, and the fat is separated out with alcohol. This method is used infrequently anymore.

Expression - also known as cold-pressing, this is a method by which essential oils are extracted from peel by pressing or breaking the peels, combining it with a minute amount of water, and soaking up the expressed oil. If you use the cold-press method on your peels, be sure the fruit has been organically grown, or the yield will include pesticide particles.

Maceration - a method by which essential oils are extracted from plants by immersion in fat and application of low heat.

Perfume - a blend of essential oils with up to about 30% essence. The fragrance of perfume lasts 4 - 6 hours, while the fragrance of cologne lasts 2 hours, and toilet water, 2 - 4 hours.

Resin Absolute - a fragrance ingredient extracted from gum resins and oleoresins by saturating them with alcohol and heating the mixture. Cassia and neroli are extracted in this way.

Resinoid - a perfume product extracted from plant exudations; that is, gums, resins, and oleoresins, by using hydrocarbon solvents. They can be solid, semi-solid, or viscous.

Skin Freshener - contains 1 part oil, 10 parts dilutant (like alcohol) and 1 part fixative.

Solvent Extraction - Method by which essential oils are extracted from a plant without having to apply high temperatures. Often hydrocarbon solvents are used in the extraction. This method has become quite popular.

Toilet Water - (also known as *Eau de Toilette* or *Eau de Parfum*) These alcohol-based perfumes only contain around 4% essential oils and 10 - 20% perfume mixed in a 90% alcohol base.

Blending Perfumes

Blending perfumes is an art, like cooking, painting, dancing, or writing. It would be an easier matter if the scent of a perfume equalled the sum of its parts, but it does not. A perfume depends on the interaction of ingredients, and interaction is hard to predict, even when you work with the same ingredients over and over again. Think about the unpredictability of human interaction, and you get an idea of what it is like with perfumes. Ideally, the perfect perfume blend is synergistic -- greater than the sum of its parts. And no one scent should stand out from the others. They should all combine into a perfectly harmonious bouquet.

Historically, cultures seem to go through periods of time when as a whole, they prefer certain kinds of scents. Examples include animal-like, and spicy scents (ancient Egypt) roses above all else (England under Charles II), or grassy, green, natural essences (the U.S. today). These days, no matter where we live, we need to create strong blends so they can compete with household cleaners, deodorants, hair sprays, and other environmental pollutants.

When you begin to blend a perfume you need to ask yourself several questions, including why and for whom you are blending. Climate and seasons play an important role in choosing scents. People in northern climes tend to prefer light florals, while those who live closer to the Equator often favor heavier, intoxicating blends. More often people are drawn to redolent, spicy fragrances in the winter, and lighter, airy scents in the summertime.

The phase through which a woman is passing in her menstrual cycle can also influence her choices. And the emotional and physical condition of both men and women can be a factor.

Age and sex are an additional consideration. Children often prefer fruit and spices (think of all the fruit-flavored children's lipsticks!); older people seem to like richer blends maybe because they can smell them better; women may be drawn to florals, citrusy, and grassy scents; men can lean toward wood, bark, roots, mosses, and resins.

Skin types make a difference. Usually, the darker the skin, the stronger the scent the person can tolerate.

When I perform personalized fragrance consultations, I consider my client's personality, lifestyle, and reasons for wanting the scent. I may be faced with a shy Pisces who wishes to appear more self-confident, or with a strong-minded Leo, who wants to accentuate her showman's persona. I blend different scents for people who work all day in an office than for tennis pros and long distance runners. Maybe my client wants to use this scent in meditations for honing his psychic abilities, or perhaps rather than wear it, she prefers to dab it on the light bulbs in her store to attract customers. Different concentrations and forms of scents may be required, depending on whether they are composed of perfumes, powders, unguents, bath products, sachets, potpourris, incenses, or massage oils.

Wearing Scents

Whether you are blending fragrances for personal or ritual occasions, remember that you will get the most mileage out of your scent if you wear it in layers. This means you should use the same blend in the bath as a cologne splash, sachet, perfume, moisturizing lotion, massage oil, etc. Blends are concocted to make a statement. Mixing blends usually takes away their punch, and at worst, can conflict.

Apply perfumes to your pulse points -- on the temples, behind the ears, at the throat, inside elbows and wrists, between the breasts, behind the knees, and at your ankles. During some rituals such as initiation ceremonies, the priestess will anoint the covener's third eye, nose, lips, breasts, lower abdomen, and soles of feet. One of the purposes of this ritual is to open up the covener's chakras to cosmic energy, and to seek a balance of mind, body, emotion, and spirit. (For a description of these types of rituals, see *Secrets of a Witch's Coven* and *Web of Light.*)

Making Your Own Essences

Naturally, it is easier to purchase essences than to manufacture them. However, some oils, particularly those taken from herbs, are difficult to obtain unless you prepare them yourself. Making your own oils during the proper moon phases, and instilling them with your personal energy makes them more potent. Essences can be extracted in alcohol, vegetable oil, or partly in water. For a distillation, simply immerse the plant in chemical-free water, 9 parts water to 1 part material, heat the water, and let it simmer for

5 - 10 minutes. Cool the mixture so that when the oil rises to the top you can skim it off with a cotton swab. It is said that in this way the Persians discovered rose water. As the story goes, a moat around a castle was filled with water and rose petals as part of a royal wedding ceremony. In the intense heat, the petals released their oil and formed a scum that when lifted off was found to be deliciously fragrant.

You don't even need to heat the water if you are willing to wait a couple of weeks. Just shake the bottle every day, and strain it through a filter. This kind of aromatic water works well with herbs like mint and chamomile.

Make a tincture by placing washed, dried flowers, herbs, etc., into a dark bottle filled with 190 proof alcohol, pure, rectified olive oil, sweet almond oil, or safflower oil. Use 6 parts alcohol for 1 part plant material. Shake the bottle once or twice a day for 21 days, then pour the liquid through a sieve or a coffee filter into another bottle.

Alternatively, you can make an *enfleurage*. This works best with flower petals. In a shallow pan lay an olive or mineral oil-soaked cotton cloth to which you have added 1 teaspoon of tincture of benzoin for every 3 cups of oil. Cover the cloth with petals, press with a piece of clean glass, and set the pan in the sunshine. Change the flowers daily for 7, 12, or 21 days, depending on the intensity you require. At the end of that period, remove the glass, and squeeze the oil from the cloth into a bottle.

In another method, fill an earthen jar with water and your botanical of choice. Set the jar out in the sun. As the scum forms, skim it off with a cotton swab stick, and fill a bottle with the oil. Add more plant material, and repeat the process until you have all the oil you need.

Now that you know how to extract your own essences, you may wish to check the list of fragrances used in perfumery and incense-making in Appendix I. It gives you more specific information on fragrances so you can decide what scents you may wish to distill for yourself. The list is not exhaustive, and, at any rate, you should write down your own ideas about these oils in your magical diary or herbal.

Now To Blend!

If all these provisos have made you think that you'd better leave fragrance chemistry to the experts, relax. Until the twentieth century, most perfume blending was done in the home, and the results were just as good then as now. All you need is some basic knowledge, a small cache of raw materials, including about 20 different oils, the fearless desire to experiment, the willingness to make mistakes, and a generous dollop of patience and practice.

Start modestly by blending no more than 3 oils in any one perfume. Even with these few oils, you can enhance the quintessence of the person for whom you are blending. Most ritual purposes, too, can be expressed with approximately 20 single notes (the fragrance of one specific substance).

Almost every book on fragrances I have read describes blending in musical terms. Perfumiers talk about scales of fragrances, melodies, harmonies, symphonies, top, middle and base notes -- even half-tones. I certainly haven't been able to come up with a better analogy. However, I think that sometimes all this musical vocabulary can make fragrance blending seem more complicated than it really is. You need only remember that most blends separate into three parts:

1) What you smell initially, the minute you uncap the bottle. This scent seems to evaporate quickly.

2) The more longlasting scent -- what the fragrance seems to be all about.

3) The subtle, underlying odor that enhances the longevity of the fragrance, balances all the combined scents, and keeps the initial smell from evaporating too quickly. In fragrance parlance, these are called top notes, middle notes, and base notes.

You should also understand the purposes of what are known in the trade as blenders. Blender enhancers can compose 15 - 50% of the perfume. They personalize your blend, but do not overpower it. Sandalwood is a good example of a blender enhancer.

Blender equalizers like rosewood can also compose up to 50% of the blend, but rather than affect the personality of your blend, they basically serve to smoothe it out so that no one of the other fragrances becomes overpowering. On the other hand, blender modifiers are intensely scented, and therefore, should only compose 1 - 3% of the perfume. This means that for every dram vialful of fragrance you should only use a couple of drops. Patchouly, with its strong odor and low evaporation rate is a classic example of a modifier. Obviously these scents change the blend, and also keep it from going flat.

A fixative is another important term. This fragrance material, composed of animal or vegetable matter, adds an individual flavor to a perfume, and helps stabilize and equalize the evaporation rate of the other ingredients. In musical terms, a fixative is a base note, and can compose up to 15% of a blend, but usually makes up no more than 5%. Some fixatives, like patchouly as mentioned above, are also blender modifiers. Here is a list of fixatives with the types of fragrances they best underscore:

angelica - fruity, herby;

benzoin - flowery, oriental, intoxicating;

calamus - spicy;

oakmoss - flowery, woodsy;

orris - flowery;

vetivert - herby, woodsy.

Other fixatives include: civet, musk, ambergris, castoreum, frankincense, myrrh, labdanum, storax, balsam of Peru, balsam of Tolu, sandalwood, tonka and vanilla beans, clary sage, reindeer moss, patchouly, ambrette seed, sweet woodruff, costus.

A few essences, like jasmine, rose, and ylang-ylang range over the entire perfume scale. They are fixatives, but also can be used as top notes and middle notes.

Formulas

As you become familiar with oils and their properties you will have no trouble inventing exactly the right personalized formulas for any occasion. However, when you are just beginning to sniff your way through the bewildering variety of scents that can be combined into perfumes it is comforting to have on hand a few reliable formulas. The following recipes from my personal Book of Shadows, that is, my own compilation of rituals and formulas, provide perfumes for different ritual occasions and demonstrate some harmonious ideas.

Aphrodite's Spell
(Love)
1/2 tsp. frankincense
1/2 tsp. Oriental musk
1/2 tsp. jasmine
1/4 tsp. honeysuckle
1/2 tsp. white rose
2 drops lavender

Gypsies' Gold
(Prosperity)
2 tsp. frankincense
1 tsp. rose
1/2 tsp. dark musk
6 drops patchouly
1/2 tsp. cyclamen
2 drops bitter almond

Helios
(Better Health)
2 tsp. heliotrope
1 tsp bayberry
4 drops geranium rose
2 drops melissa
6 drops carnation
3 drops lime
1/2 tsp. narcissus

Pentagram
(Protection)
1 tsp. red rose
1 tsp. myrrh
1 tsp. gardenia
4 drops lemon verbena

High Conquering
(Legal Aid)
1 tsp. frankincense
1/2 tsp. bay
1/2 tsp. cinnamon
6 drops Siberian fir
1 drop geranium
1/2 tsp. rose
2 tsp. jojoba oil in which you
have soaked a jalap root

Anointing
(for third eye, candles, etc.)
6 drops English lavender
1/2 tsp. carnation
1/2 tsp. citrus
1/2 tsp. lily-of-the-valley

Consecration
(for ritual instruments)
1/4 tsp. benzoin
1 tsp. olibanum
1 tsp. rose
1 tsp. lily
3 drops rosemary
1/4 tsp. carnation

Cernunnos
(invokes the Horned God)
1 tsp. amber
1/4 tsp. ambergris
1 tsp. dark musk
1/2 tsp. Indian patchouly
1/2 tsp. wild rose

Green Goddess	**Enchanted Forest**
(invokes the goddess of the field, forest, and meadow)	(invokes the Elementals)
1 tsp. daisy	1 tsp. spruce
1/2 tsp. daphne	1/2 tsp. heather
1 tsp. tea rose	1/4 tsp. opoponax
1 tsp. sandalwood	1/2 tsp. balsam fir
	1/4 tsp. fougere
	1/2 tsp. wood bouquet

Inner - Outer Beauty Spell

The far-reaching, psychological effects of essences are not to be underestimated. When appropriately worn, perfumes can increase self-awareness, bolster self-confidence, open the mind to the higher planes, and balance the personality. The Inner - Outer Beauty Spell helps accomplish these goals, integrate the personality, and strengthen the character so that the Witch can be in the best position possible to help others—which is one of our commitments as Pagans.

In this ritual you will invoke the power of the forces of Tiphareth, the central Sephira on the Qabalistic Tree of Life, which symbolizes the Divine Plan made manifest as it should be. In the balance of forces found in Tipareth resides the meaning of true beauty.

Items Required

1. A small, unpainted wooden box, which you can purchase at a craft store. If possible, try to get a box with a rounded top that opens and closes on hinges, and looks something like a tiny trunk or mini-treasure chest.

2. Acrylic paints and brush. Depending on the symbolism that is most important to you, you can paint your box heather-colored or slate blue for Virgo, or amber, yellow, or gold for the sun. Use a dark brown color to paint the symbols on the outside of the box These might include the zodiac sign for Virgo (figure 2.1), your own zodiac sign, the symbol of the Sun (figure 2.2), and sigil of Raphael (figure 2.3), Archangel of healing.

Figure 2.1
Virgo

Figure 2.2
The Sun

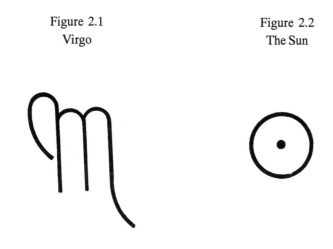

Figure 2.3
Seal of Raphael

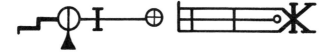

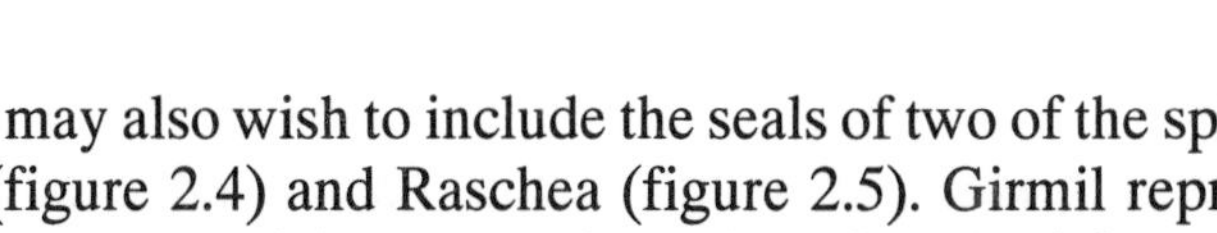

You may also wish to include the seals of two of the spirits of Girmil (figure 2.4) and Raschea (figure 2.5). Girmil represents love, harmony and beauty and teaches the Magician to love everything. (Imagine how difficult this is!) Raschea is the king of flowers, and by extension, aromatherapy. On the inside of the box top paint the Eye of Horus (figure 2.6), Egyptian symbol of protection, good luck, and well-being.

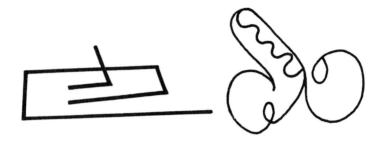

Figure 2.4
Seal of Girmil

Figure 2.5
Seal of Raschea

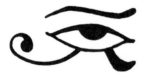

Figure 2.6
Eye of Horus

Contemplate this symbol to help open your mind to the higher realms.

You may wish to paint other personal symbols on the outside of the box, which is your prerogative. Only the Eye of Horus is necessary, but you may paint on any other symbols that are meaningful to you, especially those associated with health and protection. Prepare the box a few days before performing the ritual in order to give the paint time to dry.

3. Two white altar candles and candleholders.

4. Altar cloth in gold (for Tiphareth) or slate-blue (for Virgo).

5. Gemstones: quartz and carnelian. You will anoint these stones during the ritual and place them in the box. By tradition, quartz is thought to possess the capacity to capture and imprison illness and negativity in the voids between the crystals which form its structure. Carnelian is chosen because it is alleged by gem healers to be the ideal healing stone. Also it is under the rulership of both Virgo (beauty, health) and Leo (the healing power of the sun).

6. Anointing oils:

a. *Self-Blessing perfume* (10 drops cedar, 1 tsp. rose, 1 drop lemongrass, 6 drops benzoin).

b. *Invocation perfume* for the candles (equal parts frankincense and myrrh, 6 drops sandalwood).

c. *Horus perfume* for the Eye of Horus (1/2 tsp. frankincense, 1 tsp. rose, 3 drops lemongrass, 8 drops saffron, 4 drops cedar).

d. *Virgo perfume* for both the box and the carnelian (1 tsp. narcissus, 1/4 tsp. hyacinth, 1/2 tsp. muguet, 1/2 tsp. heliotrope, 2 tsp. sandalwood).

e. *Wings of Healing perfume* for the quartz (1/2 tsp. violet, 1/2 tsp. heliotrope, 1/2 tsp. rose.

7. Incense burner, coals and matches. Make the incense from 1 Tbs. benzoin, 1/2 tsp. crushed rose petals, 1 tsp. white sandalwood powder, 4 Tbs. yellow incense base, and 1/2 tsp. rose oil.

Preliminaries

Perform this ritual on or just after the new moon when the moon is in Virgo. Ideally, dawn is the best time, but failing that, any time in the morning before 11:00 a.m. is acceptable.

Erect your altar in the East. Take a purification bath to which you have added 1 Tbs. rosemary essence. Don a white robe or perform the ritual skyclad (in the nude).

Anoint the altar candles with Invocation perfume. First wash the candles, buff them dry with a soft cloth, and trim the wicks if necessary. Be sure that no impurities are in the wax. Beeswax candles are perfect.

Hold one candle between your palms and let it grow warm from your hands. Then breathe on it three times to instill it with the breath of life. Keep the candle in the hand you use least and anoint with the fingers of the hand you use most. Start in the middle of the candle, working your fingers all around it to the top. Returning to the middle, work your way downward to the bottom. Repeat the procedure with the other candle. When you are through, affix the candles in the holders, and place them on top of the altar cloth on either side of the altar toward the back.

Next place the incense burner on the front left corner of the altar along with the coal and incense. Keep the matches nearby, but not on the altar. The components of matches fall under the rulership of Mars, and for this ritual you do not want to invoke this influence.

Place the painted box on the center of the altar with the stones outside and in front of it. At the right front corner of the altar position your anointing oils. At the very front and center of the altar just behind your Athame, position bowls of consecrated salt and water. If you do not know how to consecrate salt and water, I direct you to *Web of Light*. [3]

The Ritual

Light the candles and incense, and meditate on the following description of Tiphareth from *A Practical Guide to Qabalistic Symbolism* by Gareth Knight:

Tiphareth represents the goal to which all must attain that Its Virtue is that of Devotion to the Great Work ... The colours of the Sephirah are pinks, yellows, and ambers which can be best perceived in the supreme beauties of the horizon at sunset and dawn. The Name of God in this Sephirah is Jehovah Aloah va Daath, meaning God Made Manifest in the Sphere of the Mind... Harmony, or Beauty, implies health and healing and so Raphael, the Archangel `which standeth in the Sun' is obviously an integral part of Tiphareth. In ritual working he is the Archangel who guards the Eastern quarter which is the quarter of the Element of Air ... also a symbol of the Spirit, free-moving and unconfined, penetrating everywhere.

Raphael can be visualized, as an alternative to the Sephirothic colours, in the colours of gold and blue of the shining disc of the sun in a clear sky, raying the healing and sustaining powers of sunlight, which include the forces of radiant heat, infra-red and ultra-violet besides the spiritual enlightenment and quickening of life of the Sun behind the Sun. He can be pictured with wings which fan the air causing a rush of fire and air which revitalises the forces of any aura it contacts it is a great contact of healing, spiritual and psychological as well as physical ... The right form of dedication is to retain all the human characteristics and yet to live a life entirely directed by principle ... This is the real function of the magician, to construct the right forms out of his own being for his own spiritual force to indwell. The ritual workings of ceremonial magic are but a special technique for raising a particular potency of life to the nthe degree to give a correct orientation to it. The real ritual is a twentyfour hours a day process of living out life according to spiritual principles so that by this talismanic action, patterns of right living are formed in the unconscious mind of the race so that this right way of living becomes easier for those who follow after." [4]

When you are ready, take your Athame, stand in the East, and perform the Lesser Banishing and Invoking Pentagram rituals.

Once you have opened the Circle, return to the East and speak the following invocations aloud:

"Raphael, god as healer, you who pause on your wind-swept mountain peak with saffron robes whirling about your lithe form, your sparkling wand held high, step swiftly from your supernal realm and pierce this Circle of Light. Quicken my understanding of true beauty so that I may devote myself to the Great Work, and in so doing, bring the vision of the harmony of all things to others.

"Virgin of the Earth, you who are immaculate as the inception of life, whose purity dissolves all negativity and imbalance, and so, subtly heals the world, caress my cheek and stay in my heart so that I may radiate your energy to the benefit of humankind."

Pause a few moments and feel the powers of Raphael and Virgo surge through your body, cleansing and purifying you. You may wish to add more incense to the hot coal at this time.

Next perform the Middle Pillar Ritual. [5] After the last part of the ritual when you visualize the white light spiralling around

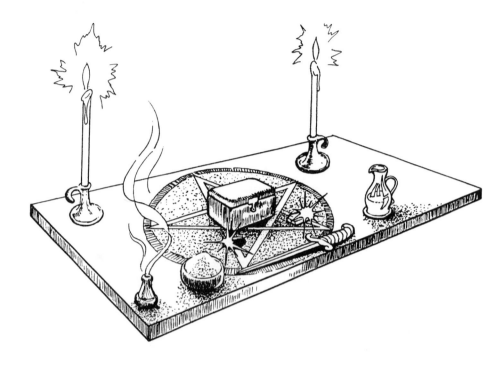

Figure 2.7
Altar for Inner-Outer Beauty Spell

you, switch focus. Imagine a ray of golden light edged with rose and amber filtering out of the cosmos and penetrating your heart chakra. Intone several times "Jehovah Aloah ve Daath"

See your entire being bathed in the golden light. You are at one with the sun. The all-encompassing, luminescent love of the deity flames around you. Bask in the light for a few minutes; experience the joy of absolute love, and remember it. When you are called upon to administer to others you will need to evoke this reservoir of love to help the healing process.

Now take the Self-Blessing oil and anoint yourself with your forefinger in the following places and say:

"Bless me, Lord and Lady, for I am your Child.

Bless my eyes that I may see the paths open to me (anoint your closed eyelids).

Bless my nose that I may inhale the essence of life and love and embody these principles (anoint the tip of your nose).

Bless my mouth that I may communicate your holy message to others (anoint your lips).

Bless my heart that I may learn to love all life and keep the Word within (anoint your heart chakra).

Bless my hands that they may be the vehicles of your power (anoint the center of each palm).

Bless my loins which manifest human life as you have brought forth all Creation (anoint your loins).

Bless my feet that I may follow your path and journey to the fulfillment of my potential in accordance with the Divine Will (anoint the center of each sole)."

You are ready to anoint the box with the Wings of Healing oil. Dab oil in the upper left corner, upper right corner, and middle of the bottom of the front side of the box (points A, B, and C). Connect points A and B. Then stroke down from the upper left corner to the bottom middle (point C), and then from the upper right corner to the point at the center of the bottom (point C again, see figure 2.8) This triangle attracts the power of the Sephirah to the box. Repeat the procedure on each exterior and interior side of the box, totalling twelve sides in all (exterior front, exterior back, exterior left side, exterior right side, exterior top, exterior bottom, interior front, interior back, interior left side, interior right side, interior top, interior bottom).

Note well: If you ever wish to repel rather than attract energy, reverse the procedure. (See figure 2.8).

Anoint the Eye of Horus symbol next. Dab Horus oil on each of the four corners of the symbol, and trace an unbroken line from the upper right corner down, and around and up again to join again at the upper right corner where you started.

Finally, prepare your stones by first dipping them in salt, then in water. Dry and anoint them with the appropriate oils (see 6. d. and e. above) and place them in the box. As time goes by, you will probably want to add other stones to the box, either to help you

Figure 2.8
How to Attract and Repel Energy with Anointing Oil

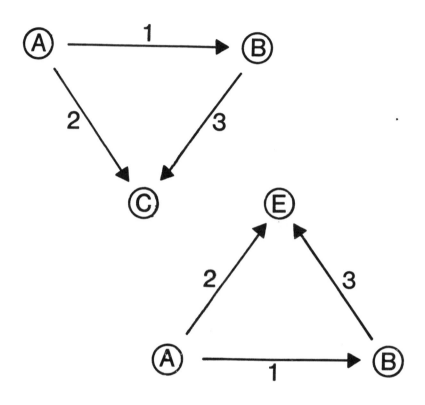

heal others and/or yourself (refer to chapter 5 in my book *Green Magic* on stone symbolism). Each time you add a new stone, perform the ritual as written above, except you will not necessarily need to do the ceremony when the moon is in Virgo, nor do you need to reconsecrate the box and Eye of Horus.

Use your box as a tool to bring you tranquility in times of trouble by opening it, taking out the stones and lining them up in front of the box. Then meditate on the Eye of Horus. Use the box in the same way to put yourself in the proper frame of mind when you are called upon to aid others -- inside is contained all the healing power of Divine Love.

Close the Circle by performing the Lesser Banishing Pentagram Ritual, and thank the spirits and particularly the Virgin Goddess and the Healer Archangel Raphael for lending you their power and protection. The rite is ended. Blessed Be!

You may wish to keep in your box a number of dram vials filled with healing oils. I recommend any of the following: apple blossom, chamomile, basil, geranium, lily-of-the-valley, benzoin, civet (for magnetism), iris, Siberian fir, pine, sweet pea, violet, primrose, and rose. Choose other oils according to the information given in Appendix I.

Chapter 3:

Bathing Beauty
A Short History of Bathing

Although washing may have felt good to primitive people, early cultures probably did not associate immersion in water with cleanliness and healthiness. People undoubtedly only bathed in lakes and streams when they happened upon them, and it was convenient, and the weather was not too cold. Bathing as we know it only became possible when societies stabilized enough to haul water from its source to the tub. At first, this activity was carried out by slaves with pails, then by pipes. The oldest known bathroom, ascertained to be 6,000 years old, is in India. Ancient engineers' undoubted skills at designing pipelines and sewer systems are attested to by the 1,500-year-old toilets and sewers in Mesopotamia that still transmit water today.

Egyptians, as in many other realms, dominated ancient bathing practices. They even took showers! Nonetheless, the art of bathing in early times did not reach its "highwater mark" until the Roman era when personal hygiene enjoyed a heyday. For example, the baths at Caracalla, built in 217 A.D., could hold up to 18,000 bathers at one time. Roman baths constituted small towns unto themselves, often sporting game rooms, libraries, art galleries, meeting rooms, and temples, as well as the more mundane cold and hot water therapy baths and exercise rooms which many of us enjoy today at our health clubs. A far cry from splashing around in a six-foot tub with a rubber duckie!

Nothing remains static, however. Along with the breakdown of morals in Roman society mixed bathing houses began to predominate, and eventually many establishments degenerated into brothels. After the fall of Rome, these dens of depravity were singled out as characteristic of the Romans' sybaritic, wicked lifestyle, and bathing as a whole was condemned as contributing to moral degradation.

Although bathing made a brief comeback in Europe when the Crusaders returned from the East imbued with Oriental ideas of cleanliness, the reputation of bath houses, known as stews, and dens of gaming, prostitution, and other vices, persisted. Finally, under the dictates of the Church the stews were shut down.

Several centuries passed during which Europeans generally felt it immodest and unhealthy to wash at all. Many women, for example, bathed only twice in their lives, once at birth, and again at marriage. Even our Puritan forefathers believed that bathing promoted promiscuity. For instance, in Philadelphia, a person could be thrown in jail for taking more than one bath a month!

Attitudes toward bathing altered under the influence of the Victorians, who believed that "cleanliness was next to godliness." Over my own lifetime I can see how notions have changed because I remember how as a little girl I only took one full bath a week, usually on Saturday night.

Throughout the latter part of the last century and into the twentieth, the quality and quantity of bathrooms has kept improving so that nowadays it is not unusual to find American homes built with bedroom-size bathrooms complete with gigantic soaking tub, showers with several heads, jacuzzi, hot tub, sauna, entertainment center, and lounge chairs. It has been quipped that when archeologists from some future century uncover the remains of contemporary America, we will be known for our bathrooms.

Why Take a Bath?

Because it helps us clean, disinfect, and maintain our skin, which with an average 3,000 square inches, is twice the weight of either our livers or brains, and makes our skin the largest organ of our bodies. Skin protects us from pollution and other injuries, helps us breathe, excretes toxins, regulates our internal temperature, and with seventy-two feet of nerves per square inch, provides us with strong sensory stimuli. With all that going for it, I think our skin deserves a little extra attention!

Soaking in warm water helps sluff off dead, decaying cells so that the pores do not become clogged and cease to function. Epsom or sea salts especially draw toxins from the body. Baths relax and soothe tired, sore muscles, and calm the nerves. With the proper water temperature and appropriate bath oils you can also soften and rejuvenate your skin, stimulate your circulation, and maybe even enjoy yourself. I know a romance novel writer who claims to do her best creative work in the tub!

Bathing and Magic

If you have read many books about the Craft, you may have noticed that in Wicca we take a lot of baths, usually before performing most spells or rituals except, perhaps, morning meditation. We bathe to purify ourselves symbolically because we believe that when we enter the Circle we leave all our flaws outside in the mundane world and for the period of time spent within that sacred space, we become perfect beings.

In this practice Witches are not alone. Let me share a couple of illustrations from the Brazilian neo-African religion known as Macumba. One of Macumba's most popular deities is the sea goddess Iemanjá. Her sacred day is celebrated on December 31 in Rio de Janeiro. On that evening everyone migrates to the beach and lights candles and fires in honor of the goddess. At midnight as the firecrackers erupt from atop the roofs of the luxury hotels raucously proclaiming the New Year, the faithful gather below and quietly send out little boats into the open water laden with gifts for the Mistress of the Sea. Many people wade in and take ritual baths to show their devotion.

When I lived in Brazil, I witnessed this and similar ceremonies. One day shortly before the celebration I was sitting on the beach with some university colleagues. One of our group was a devout Marxist with whom I had often engaged in lively political discussions. I noticed that my friend had brought two small pails with him and that he filled up one with sand and the other with water, and took them to his car.

"Celso," I asked when he returned, "what did you do that for?"

"It happens that I am going to be away in the interior of the country on New Year's Eve," he replied. "It will be the first Iemanjá Day ever that I'll spend away from the beach. So I think that at midnight I'll dump the sand on the ground and stand barefoot in it and pour the bucket of water over my head as a substitute for bathing in the ocean. In that way, no evil will befall me in the New Year."

I couldn't believe my ears. "I thought as a Marxist you didn't go in for all that stuff?"

He smiled. "But I'm a Brazilian Marxist, and I believe it doesn't hurt to cover all my bases."

Another time I had the good fortune to be invited to join in one of the private rituals of some Macumba practitioners as if I were an initiate. They extended to me this courtesy because I was a Wicca Priestess, but even so, I had to be purified before I could participate.

I was led to a tiny bathroom -- not more than a shower stall -- by two handmaidens. They stripped me of my clothes and poured over my head two pitchers of a mixture of fragrant herbs, oils, and water, and let the residue drip to the floor. I was glad the outdoor temperature was about 100 degrees Fahrenheit or I would have frozen before I air-dried. As it was, I felt pleasantly refreshed by this herbal bath the Macumbeiros call an *amaci*.

The women dressed me in the style of the entity which they determined watched over me, wound my head in a turban, and festooned me with silver jewelry. At last, I was ready to take part in the secret rite ... which unfortunately must remain untold!

The point of these stories is to show that purification bathing is a key element of most religions, whether the participants be Southern Baptists, Brazilian Macumbeiros, or Celtic Witches.

When I was first studying Wicca, long before I thought that I might want to be initiated into the Craft, I experienced a memorable dream. I sat nude, outdoors in a pine-scented forest under a star-embroidered sky immersed in a bathtub filled to the brim with crystals of fragrant rose water. Several women attended me in my ablutions. It seemed that every time the water cascaded over me from their hands I was being covered by scintillating stardust. My entire body thrilled to the flow of the water, and I felt dazzled by radiant cosmic love.

The dream impressed me so much I wrote to my teacher, Lady Sara Cunningham-Carter. She told me that I had experienced an initiation dream, and that such occurrences were common right before or just after a Witch was inducted into the Craft. I can only hope that each one of you who decide to follow the gentle path of Wicca will experience such a dream. The incident helped me understand that what we strive for in the Craft is not impossible, nor is it a figment of our imaginations. Unity with a superintelligence composed of boundless love is an attainable reality.

Taking a Bath

Whether you bathe for ritual purposes or just to relax, I usually recommend taking a warm bath (90 - 98 degrees Fahrenheit). Hot baths (up to 115 degrees) can be enervating, and should be followed by a cool shower to bring the body's temperature back to normal. If you are a woman, never take a hot bath (or get into a jacuzzi or hot tub) when you are pregnant. Cool baths (down to 78 degrees) are invigorating and soothe tender skin smarting from sunburn or a rash, but they should be followed by warm showers to normalize the body's temperature.

Once or twice a week when you have a half an hour's time, draw a warm bath. While you are waiting for the tub to fill, lay out everything you need from bath salts to skin emollients, bath pillow for your head and neck, towels, etc. Moisten two cotton balls with an infusion of chamomile tea or witch hazel to place over your closed eyes. Take a quick shower to remove surface dirt and cosmetics, and rub the rough spots on your elbows, knees and heels with sweet almond oil or apricot kernel oil. Drop in the salts, crystals, or bath bag of your choice while the tub is filling. At last, you are ready to step in and luxuriate.

After bathing, rub yourself briskly with a towel until dry, and apply emollients to your face and body. This is a perfect time to give yourself a manicure or pedicure, as your nails and cuticles are softer after bathing.

You can take many kinds of baths including herbal, salts, mineral, oil, vinegar, steam, sauna, sitz, whirlpool, aromatherapy, sand, sea, milk, or sun and moon baths (see the end of this chapter for these two special ritual baths). Whichever you try you will find it a rewarding experience.

Bath Products

Originally, bath salts and crystals were meant to soften water and add fragrance. Bubble bath added fragrance and foam, and oils reduced the water's drying action and relieved itching due to skin aging and low humidity. Nowadays, commercially produced salts, crystals, bubble baths, and oils may perform several of these functions. The most common bath additives are salts, which are easily obtainable at the grocery or drugstore. Purchase rock salt, Epsom salts, borax, or washing soda, and cornstarch to soften the skin. Mix in a few drops of essential oils and food coloring to make them pretty and tint the bath water.

For effervescent salts Louise Gruenberg in *Potpourri: The Art of Fragrance Crafting* [6] recommends mixing 10 parts cream of tartar with 9 parts baking soda and 6 parts rice flour or arrowroot starch, and 1 part essential oil.

I call my favorite all-around salts recipe to which I add different oils, coloring and botanicals "Basic Salts."

Basic Salts Recipe
1 cup Epsom salts
3 teaspoons cornstarch
1 teaspoon baking powder

Blend together all the ingredients. This recipe is easy to mix, takes additives well, and does not dry out the skin. Add the oils and 1/2 - 1 tsp. food coloring depending on how intensely you want to color the water. Sometimes I include small amounts of botanicals like lavender, rosebuds, or chamomile flowers to add interest and increase the magical and beautifying virtues of the blend. I never put in so many botanicals that I make it hard to clean out the tub or clog the drain.

In the classes I teach on aromatherapy, I have found that this recipe presents students with an alternative way to experiment with blending oils. Sometimes when they combine several essential oils in a dram vial and sniff the results, then repeat the process over and over again, the combination of fragrances can overpower. Instead, if they blend the same amount of oils into the basic bath salts medium, the fragrance is somewhat absorbed, and becomes less overwhelming, but no less true. The students take home the salts and sprinkle them in the tub. Rather than having to form an opinion about the blend on the spot in the laboratory where many fragrances are competing for attention, they can take their time to sniff the recipe as it disperses in the steam and see how it combines with their skins.

Here are some salts recipes for different ritual occasions. They all begin with the basic blend to which the oils, botanicals, and coloring are added.

Dragonbane (Countermagic)

1 tsp. rose, 1 tsp. amber, 1 tsp. jasmine, 1 tsp. dark musk, 1 bay leaf crushed, 1/2 tsp. rue herb, red coloring.

Concentration (Mental Clarity)

1/4 tsp. cinnamon, 4 drops clary sage, 1/4 tsp. Siberian fir, 1/2 tsp. civet, 1 tsp. carnation, 1 tsp. lotus blossom, 1/2 tsp. heather, orange coloring.

Egyptian Sun (Energizer)

1 tsp. lotus oil, 12 drops lemongrass, 1/2 tsp. myrrh, 1/4 tsp. juniper, 1/2 tsp. bergamot, 1 tsp. crushed lemongrass herb, pinch marjoram herb, yellow coloring.

Invocation

1/2 tsp. parvati sandalwood, 1 tsp. frankincense, 1 tsp. myrrh, 1/4 tsp. allspice, 1 tsp. whole cloves, bruised, violet coloring.

Love

1 tsp. amber, 1/2 tsp. light musk, 1 tsp. rosewood, 1/2 tsp. lime, 1/4 tsp. Singapore patchouly, pinch of patchouly leaves, pink coloring.

Meditation

1/2 tsp. sandalwood, 1 tsp. hyacinth, 1-1/2 tsp. Oriental musk, 1/2 tsp. peony, 1 tsp. acacia flowers, no coloring.

Inner Temple (Peace and Harmony)

1 tsp. sandalwood, 1/2 tsp. frankincense, 1 tsp. rose, 4 drops lavender, 1/2 tsp. mignonette, blue coloring.

Sweet Dreams (Tranquil Sleep)

1 tsp. violet, 1/2 tsp. narcissus, 1/2 tsp. muguet, 1 tsp. damask rose, 6 drops labdanum, 1 tsp. chamomile flowers, 1/2 tsp. valerian herb, light green coloring.

Bath Bags

If you have never tried using a bath bag in the tub you are in for a rare treat. These herbal delights are composed of dried or fresh botanicals, oatmeal, and/or bran, ground almonds or myrrh, and sometimes soap chips and essential oils. The best part is that if you do not have the time or inclination to take a proper bath you can hang the bag from the showerhead and achieve some of the same effect. Also, you can simmer a handful of botanicals in two quarts of boiling water for 15 - 20 minutes, strain, and add the herbal water and some essential oils to your bath. For an invigorating bath, steep the botanicals in the same amount of vinegar, or if your skin needs extra attention, in milk.

If you opt for a bag, make it from muslin or cheesecloth because the porous material really lets the oils seep through. Cut enough material to make a three- to four-inch square, which you can tie together with a string or ribbon after you have filled it. Before you get out of the tub, rub yourself all over with the outside of the bag. Sometimes you can reuse a bath bag, especially if you include lots of peels, seeds, and bark, all of which release their oils slowly. If you do not use oatmeal, bran, or another meal you can simmer the contents of a spent bag in hot water on the stove like a potpourri to really exhaust the contents. When the botanicals are spent, add them to the garden soil as mulch, and refill the bag.

Typical Bath Bag Botanicals

acacia flowers (dry skin)
basil (facial steam)
blackberry leaves (stimulant)
borage (drawing)
burdock (oily skin; facial steam)
calamus (itchy skin; avoid when pregnant)
calendula (itchy skin)
cedar granules (antiseptic; avoid when pregnant)

citron (oily skin)
clary sage (euphoric)
cleaver's herb (sunburn)
clover (dry skin; facial steam)
comfrey (aging skin; facial steam)
coriander seed (stress reliever)
elder flowers (softener)
eucalyptus (sore muscles)
fennel seed (dry skin; stimulant; facial steam)
geranium (antiseptic; mild tranquilizer)
hops (tranquilizer)
horsetail (oily skin; facial steam)
Irish moss (softener; nourisher)
juniper berries (stimulant; acne cure)
kelp (softener; nourisher)
lady's mantle (freckle remover)
lavender flowers (oily skin)
lemon balm (skin tonic)
lemongrass (dry skin; cure for lice)
lemon peel (tightener)
linden flowers (skin smoother; facial steam)
lovage (soother; lessens wrinkles)
maidenhair fern (soother)
marigold flowers (oily skin)
nettles (astringent)
orange blossom (dry skin; deodorant)
parsley (oily skin; add to facial steam)
pine needles (skin refresher; rubefacient)
rose buds, hips, petals (oily skin; astringent; facial beautifier)
Roman chamomile (dry skin; add to facial steam)
rosemary (oily skin; improves capillary action)
sage (oily skin; helps cure sores; stimulant; aids conception)
sandalwood chips (acne cure)
Solomon's seal (skin abrasions)
spearmint leaves (oily skin, refreshing)
strawberry leaves (dry skin; tightens pores in facial steam)
thyme (oily skin; fights infections)
uva ursi (oily skin; female problems)
verbena (restorer for postoperative baths when permitted)
vetivert (nervous exhaustion)

violet (dry skin; facial steam)
witch hazel (skin toner and energizer)
yarrow (oily skin)
yellow dock (helps cure chronic skin diseases)

Bath Bag Recipes

These recipes will give you ideas on how to fill your own bags. Obviously, the combinations are almost endless; so I suggest you treat these formulas merely as guidelines. Refer to Appendix I in this book and the herbal chapter of my book, *Green Magic* to find other ingredients. Make sure the oatmeal is old-fashioned oats, not quick oats, or you will end up with a soggy mess.

Ishtar Bath Bag
1 cup oatmeal, 2 cups rose petals, 1 cup damiana, 1/2 cup orange blossoms, 1/2 cup orange peel, 1 cup linden flowers, 1 cup acacia flowers, 1/4 cup oak bark, 2 Tbs. jasmine oil, 2 Tbs. Oriental musk oil, 1 tsp. clove oil, 2 tsp. bergamot oil

Alpine Meadow Bath Bag
1 cup oatmeal, 1/4 cup thyme, 1/2 cup life everlasting flowers, 1/2 cup rose petals, 1/4 cup cornflowers, 1/2 cup clover tops, 1/4 cup lemon balm, 2 Tbs. sweet woodruff, 2 Tbs. sage, 1 Tbs. marjoram, 2 Tbs. green herbal oil, 2 Tbs. heather oil, 1 Tbs. carnation oil, 2 tsp. apple blossom oil, 1 tsp. geranium oil, 1 tsp. heather oil

Cloud 9 Bath Bag
1 cup oats, 1 cup elder flowers, 1/4 cup saffron, 1/2 cup lemon verbena, 1 Tbs. life everlasting flowers, 1/4 cup crushed balm of Gilead buds (poplar), 1/4 cup orange or lemon peel, 1 Tbs. carnation oil, 2 tsp. clover oil, 2 tsp. bergamot oil, 2 tsp. rose oil, 1 tsp. frankincense oil

Serenity Bath Bag
1 cup oatmeal, 1/2 cup rosemary leaves, 1/4 cup hops, 1/2 cup lavender flowers, 1 cup Roman chamomile flowers, 1/4 cup linden, 2 Tbs. valerian, 2 Tbs. rose oil, 2 Tbs. jasmine oil, 1 Tbs. lily-of-the-valley oil.

Other epidermal-friendly additives for the bath include cream, skim milk, honey, finely ground almond meal, barley, bran, oatmeal, crushed strawberries, beer, and white wine. In the same way these ingredients sustain the body from the inside they can also feed it from the outside. And if you think that any of these products seem like faddish piffle, consider that recipes for herbal and vapor baths concocted with honey, vinegar, milk, ale, and even butter have been around since the era of the Old English Herbals.

You can invent a superior shower gel based on aloe vera, which already is a gel. Add 15-20 drops of essential oils to 4 oz. of gel.

Since alcohol dries out the skin, a healthier aftershave can be whipped up from witch hazel and a few drops of essential oils. To invent a skin freshener for the entire body, blend 10 parts witch hazel, 1 part fixative (I like to use tincture of benzoin) and 1 part essential oil. Formulate a safe, talcum-type bath powder from cornstarch or arrowroot plus a few drops of essential oil.

Especially during the winter you may prefer a super-moisturizing bath oil. To 1 quart of vegetable oil (see descriptions below) add 1/4 pound of crushed botanicals. Make sure the herbs are entirely covered with oil or they may moulder. Shake the bottle every day for a week, then strain out the oil through a piece of cheesecloth. Add essential oils, and you end up with a quart of bath oil. One or two tablespoons should be enough for each bath.

Massage Oils

A chapter on the bath would not be complete without a few recipes for massage oils. Therapeutic and sexual use of massage oils is one of the kindest gifts you can bestow on your body. Massage aids your magical development because it helps balance you physically and mentally.

To every 4 oz. of massage oil I usually add 1 teaspoon vitamin E oil and 1/2 tsp. wheat germ oil. This makes a basic oil that helps stabilize and preserve the blend and feeds the skin. Here are some base oils you can use both for massage and in the bath. They all help the skin to breathe and protect it from the elements. These oils can also be used to extend a perfume blend. Following are some recipes for your enjoyment.

Base Oils

Aloe vera - derived from a desert plant, this oil tightens sagging skin and heals epidermal injuries, skin allergies, psoriasis, and eczema.

Sweet almond - a basic, light massage oil that has been used to beautify the skin since Roman times. It used to be inexpensive, but due to a recent crop failure, the wholesale price has more than doubled.

Apricot kernel - a general, edible skin conditioner.

Avocado - this oil nourishes and restores the skin. It is high in vitamins.

Borage - fortifies skin cells and protects. It is a good oil for those who live in a highly polluted environment, like a big city. Unfortunately, it needs refrigeration.

Cocoa butter - an emollient that is solid at room temperature. It is well known as a suntan lotion ingredient.

Evening primrose - although this oil makes a superior skin nourisher, it is expensive and needs refrigeration.

Grapeseed - a cleanser and toner for oily skin. Since the wholesale price of the oil is inexpensive, it is becoming an increasingly popular commercial massage oil base.

Hazelnut - this oil is widely used in skin care products like lipstick, cold creams, and lotions because it heals damaged skin.

Jojoba - this expensive product is rendered from the fruit of a 10-foot tall desert plant. It is excellent for skin infections and helps make suntans last longer. Because of its very long shelf life it is the perfect perfume diluter.

Olive - a disinfectant, wound healer and emollient. However, some people object to its strong odor.

Rapeseed - a light, odorless oil also known as Canadian oil or canola oil. It penetrates the skin easily and stays fresh for a long time.

Rosa moschata - this Chilean rosehip oil is a good emollient and tissue restorer.

Sesame -protects against the sun's harmful rays. Take care to buy the cold-pressed kind that contains the antioxidants.

Wheat germ - an edible antioxidant oil high in vitamins E, A, D and lecithin. Add a few drops to massage oils as a fortifier. But don't use too much or you will not be able to overcome the strong odor.

Massage Oil Recipes

Ishtar
(sensual)
4 oz. basic oil
1 tsp. Oriental musk
1 tsp. jasmine
1/2 tsp. floral spice
1 tsp. dark musk
1/4 tsp. clove or allspice

Cloud 9 (euphoric)
4 oz. basic oil
1 tsp. carnation
1/2 tsp. sweet clover
1/2 tsp. rose
1/2 tsp. Scotch broom
1/4 tsp. bergamot
1/2 tsp. frankincense

Ultra
(sports - helps keep
environmental pollutants from
penetrating the skin)
4 oz. basic oil
1 tsp. eucalyptus
1/4 tsp. basil
1/4 tsp. juniper
1/4 tsp. marjoram
1/2 tsp sage
1/2 tsp. bay
1/2 tsp. chypre

Mountain Meadow
(refreshing)
4 oz. basic oil
1 tsp. green herbal
1 tsp. fougere
1 tsp. heather
1/2 tsp. cornflower

Cadiz Musk
(sensual)
4 oz. basic oil
1 tsp. dark musk
1 tsp. light musk
1/2 tsp. carnation

Earth Magic
(earthy sensual)
4 oz. basic oil
2 tsp. rose
1 tsp. civet
1 tsp. blue lilac
1/2 tsp. patchouly

Heavenly Body Baths

Unusual kinds of "baths" that you will not find in a country herbal are moon and sun "baths" for magical self-development. My priestess, Lady Sara, gives a recipe for the classic Moon Bath in her *Book of Light*.

Magnetic Moon Bath

This ritual should be performed on the night of the FULL MOON. For the best results it should be performed outdoors.

First you must make a filter out of RED glass or celluloid. It should be one foot in diameter and circular.

On the night of the Full Moon you should stand outside gazing directly at the moon. If you are a man, hold the filter in such a manner that the moon's rays pass through the filter to shine on your pelvic area. If you are a woman, then hold the filter so that the moon's rays shine on your breast area. While absorbing the moon's rays you should breathe deeply and evenly. Do this for about ten minutes, then set the filter aside and perform the MIDDLE PILLAR ritual. After the ritual remain in silent meditation for a few moments before retiring.

This Magnetic Moon bath is said to increase one's vitality and sexual potency. For best results the ritual should be performed in the nude, however, since this is not generally possible I suggest a loose robe of some sort. The material should be cotton, not nylon, silk or wool. Take off all jewelry and wrist watches as they neutralize the energy.[7]

Sun Bath

The purpose of this bath is to attune yourself to active, male solar energy. It is perfect for occasions when you feel you need to become empowered, or when you are under the weather. In this visualization you will draw the energizing power of the sun into your body through the use of incense, oils, an Egyptian invocation, and imagery.

Perform the ritual at noon on a day filled with sunshine. Go to a hilltop (or if this is not possible, a park, cheerful garden, or even the middle of your room, as long as it has a south-facing window. Plan to arrive about 15 minutes before the sun is at its zenith.

Items required: a square of gold or yellow-colored cloth about the size of a beach blanket, kyphi incense (the recipe is in chapter 4), incense burner, coals and a match, 4 solar anointing oils (bay, cyclamen, heliotrope, cinnamon), one empty dram vial and cap.

Place the cloth on the ground and the lighted coal on the incense burner. In ancient Egypt the priests burned kyphi to their gods at dawn, noon and dusk. Sprinkle incense on the lighted coal, and carry the smoking burner around the Circle, from East to South, West, and North, ending in the East. All the while chant:

"Snutri, Snutri, Snutri!"

This is the Egyptian word for "incense" and it means literally "that which makes divine."

Place the burner in the East. Add more incense if you like, and pick up the oils. Sprinkle a drop of bay on the ground in the East, cyclamen in the South, heliotrope in the West, and cinnamon in the North.

Return to the center of the cloth and transfer some of the oil from each bottle into the empty dram vial in the proportion of 1/2 part bay, 1 part cyclamen, 2 parts heliotrope, and 6 drops cinnamon. Do not worry about being exact in your measurements. Cap the vial, and shake it well.

Kneel facing South, and anoint yourself with the mixture at the third eye, solar plexus, wrists, ankles, and soles of your feet. Say,

"Urhu hekennu ma-o kua," which means, "Having anointed myself with unguents, I have made myself strong."

If you have timed the ritual right, the sun should be at its highest point in the sky. With arms outstretched above your head, call several times,

"Tua Ra" (Ra, I adore thee).

Still facing South, sit cross-legged and drink in the energizing sun's rays for a few minutes. You may wish to visualize any of the following:

1) the sun god, Ra;

2) a king clothed in saffron robes sitting on a throne with his feet resting on a globe;

3) A laughing woman standing in a chariot drawn by four dancing white horses. In her right hand she holds a looking-glass, and in her left, a staff that leans against her breast.

When you feel sufficiently empowered, clear the ritual space and leave. If you wish to offer something as a token of good will and thanks, pour some milk mixed with honey on the ground.

Chapter 4:

Through Smoke

On a recent trip to Britain, I was meandering down a cobblestone street in wet and windy Cambridge when I suddenly caught a whiff of burning incense. I couldn't tell whether the heady aroma was escaping from an open shop door or the window of a private flat. In any case, the effect was to immediately dissolve my cold discomfort and loneliness at being so far away from my sunny Colorado home. My senses were revitalized, charged with a deep feeling of well-being. This is the power of incense–to calm, excite, even reach the furthest recesses of the psyche and stimulate the imagination.

Long ago, the ancients discovered these special qualities and transformed incense into a fundamental magical tool, in much the same way that it is used in the Catholic Church today. When offering ritual sacrifices, it was soon found that some woods, like cedar and aloes, emitted fresh, pleasant scents that masked the stench of the barbecue. People quickly made the act of burning incense a way to show respect to their gods and to symbolize prayer. They named this ritual procedure *per fumen*, "through smoke," which is the origin of the word "perfume." To these primitive cultures, lighting a fire, and transmuting it into fragrant smoke, took on a highly mystical and magical significance.

The custom spread throughout the world. Celtic and Nordic tribes, Egyptians, Greeks, Arabs, and Orientals all applied incense in religious rites of invocation, evocation, purification, and offertory. For example, the Egyptians on burying their dead, burned special blends to speed the departed souls to their new destinations in the next world. Contemporary Witches maintain that incense exerts profound psychological and physical effects on the human organism. This ingrained part of ritual moves us on the deepest levels of the subconscious mind, and encourages memories from the pool of the universal unconscious to emerge to the surface of conscious thought.

Some incenses are characterized as "active." They command, attract, effect changes, drive away evil, and protect. Others are considered passive, and are burned to establish an atmosphere conducive to spirituality, serenity, sensuality, and clairvoyance. Still other incenses act as hallucinogens, and in fact, include hallucinogenic ingredients such as datura, belladonna, mandrake, hellebore, monkshood, opium poppy, etc. These dangerous herbs compose part of the Witches' Flying Ointment recipes of bygone days, which I describe in *Green Magic*. If Witches of that era actually inhaled, ingested, or smeared themselves with these concoctions, they certainly would have deluded themselves into thinking that they were empowered to fly. That is, of course assuming that the potions did not kill them first.

These days in Magic, incenses serve many purposes—meditation, increased psychic awareness, inducement of a trance state, aid to astral projection, purification, protection, Countermagic, relaxation, sleep, romantic stimulation, love, friendship, deodorization, fumigation, health, beauty, prosperity, legal aid, to cause changes of any sort, or for pure enjoyment.

Besides simply burning incense during a spell or ritual, you can use it in other creative ways. Sprinkle some on a piece of parchment on which you have drawn a sigil to activate its force. Or pass the parchment through incense smoke so that it becomes permeated with the aroma. Drop a pinch of incense on a candle flame, then make a wish. Or add a special botanical or perfume oil to a general temple incense to concentrate on a specific purpose. Before going out, pass your hands through the smoke, up and down, left to right, then back and forth to attract the influence you desire. Or hold the powder tight in your hand and throw it to the four quarters before stepping over the threshold. Finally, you can anoint your third eye with incense.

Burning Incense

When I talk about burning incense, I refer to the powdered kind, not commercially prepared incense sticks. The difference between powdered and stick incense, in my opinion, is rather like the difference between fine Darjeeling loose tea and generic supermarket tea bags. Once you try the connoiseur's choice you will never want to go back to the pedestrian brand. Powdered incense also has the advantage because you can add oils and botanicals to an already prepared formula to vary the theme, and you can use it like a sachet and sprinkle it on talismans or magical tools in Circle.

To burn powdered incense purchase special coals that are called "self-lighting" or "quick-igniting," made from willow wood and saltpeter. I advise against barbecue coals because they emit noxious fumes which present danger within the enclosed space of an indoor Circle. You need a coal because most good incense is not self-igniting. It does not contain saltpeter, which adulterates the aroma, and as a result, the magical intention. When you burn loose incense, the self-lighting coals contain the saltpeter which burns off rapidly after the coal is ignited. Add the incense to the hot coal.

To keep your coals from getting too much moisture in them, wrap them in aluminum foil and store them in an airtight box with some silica gel beads or sand mixed with borax. If moisture eventually ruins a coal, try adding a drop or two of alcohol or perfume just before lighting it.

If you are a purist, or cannot find these coals, you can make your own by crushing 12 parts of high-quality wood charcoal and adding 1 part saltpeter and a binding agent like tragacanth gum or gum arabic dissolved in some water, or egg white. Spread the mixture in a foil-lined pan and score it so that the coals will be easier to break into smaller pieces once they dry.

Purchase any cauldron-style incense burner, or a glazed clay pot with a wide mouth. If you prefer a metal burner, line it with fresh foil each time you use it so that odors from previous burnings will not cling to the sides. If you have a clay pot, fill it with sand, clean earth, small pebbles, or tiny shells to prevent the pot from cracking. If you use sand, make a few scratch marks in it to insure even burning of the coal. You can easily scoop away the ash-covered sand after each burning, and add a new layer of sand for the next time you light incense, thereby assuring clean burning without mixing aromas.

Light the coal (you may break it in half for the sake of economy, or use the smaller size coals), and place it in the incense burner. The charcoal will catch fire immediately and sizzle as the saltpeter burns off. It takes about thirty seconds for the coal to burn all the way through. Once it stops sizzling and begins to glow, spoon a small amount of incense on the hot coal. Tin, silver, or glass spoons available from head shops, specialty gourmet shops, or tobacco stores are ideal for this purpose. I use an aluminum spice scoop that looks like a Liliputian shovel.

Continue to add more incense if you wish until the coal is extinguished—for up to thirty minutes. Avoid accidents by never leaving your burner unattended when in use. After the burner cools, dispose of the ashes and foil, or remove the top layer of sand.

Incense-Making

Putting together incense is a bit like creating a potpourri or sachet, only you do not need to bother with color, texture, fixatives, and spices. Instead, concentrate on botanicals, like gums, resins, and bases, that release their fragrances when burned. With practice, you can learn to blend exotic scents from barks, spices, flowers, seeds, roots, gums, resins, woods—even from animal tissue, although I do not recommend it.

Know how to prepare your own incense so you can create a satisfying personalized scent suited to your desires and needs. If you make your own incense and are sure of the ingredients and that the incense was blended at the best astrological time, the product will be more effective for you. Blend active incenses when the moon is waxing to full, and passive incenses or incenses for Countermagic when the moon is waning. The day of the week you choose to do your blending is also influential. For example, you might put together a love incense on a Friday, or an incense to help protect you in travel on a Monday, or a recipe to sell your house on a Saturday.

Although many metaphysical supplies stores furnish high quality incense, others skimp on ingredients and use inferior oils. Some inexpensive, Far Eastern formulas actually use dung as a base, and mask the stench with cheap oils. So, let the buyer beware!

Testing Ingredients

Test incense ingredients like essential oils, only burn them and smell the smoke rather than rub them on your skin. When experimenting with materials, at first burn only a small amount, then slowly make additions until the scent becomes distinguishable from the odor of the burning coal. Do not sample more than six ingredients at a sitting, or you may overload your senses. Be sure to remove all vestiges of a previous ingredient from the glowing coal before testing another so you get the truest odor possible. In a separate notebook or your herbal, characterize the fragrances as warm or cool, light or heavy, pleasant, sharp, sensual, bitter, fetid, etc., according to the fragrance vocabulary you developed for perfumes. Also note the planetary or astrological associations of each botanical.

Many incenses are comprised primarily of frankincense, myrrh, benzoin, or sandalwood; so familiarize yourself with these ingredients first. Increase your palette by sampling cedarwood, cinnamon, copal, galbanum, balsam of Peru, balsam of Tolu, clove, bay leaves, bayberry bark, evergreen needles, juniper berries, vanilla, crushed tonka, coumarin crystals, allspice berries, poplar buds, rosemary, thyme, mint, life everlasting flowers, lemongrass, musk ambrette seed, storax, dragon's blood resin, geranium flowers, ambergris, and mastic. While not the only incense-making ingredients, they are some of the most common.

Incense Bases

For best results combine your ingredients with bases that are pre-colored or which you color yourself. First, combine your gums, resins, woods, and crushed botanicals in a mixing bowl. Add the oils and mix; then stir in the base.

Commercially prepared pre-colored and pre-scented incense bases are convenient and smooth-textured, readily absorb oils, and combine well with botanicals. However, the scents and colors often leave something to be desired. Also they are difficult to obtain unless you have a resale license or can find a retail supplier. The Delphic Oracle, 1546 - 28th St., Boulder, Colorado 80303 sells superior bases.

Those who prefer to make their own bases often use talc or a wood base. I advise against talc because breathing it in can be harmful to your lungs. Wood base is a fancy name for sawdust. If you own a saw, you can make the sawdust yourself. Alternatively, sweep it up from a woodworker's shop floor. The kind of sawdust you collect—oak, pine, alder, ash, etc. —depends on the type of ritual for which you wish to burn the incense. Some wood ingredients are listed in Appendix I, but in *Web of Light* I include a comprehensive treatment of tree symbolism.

To custom-design your own colors try the following:

green: benzoin, spruce needles, green juniper berries, moss, storax.

red: grains of paradise, scarlet balm, red geranium flowers, ambergris.

blue: violet and red bases, violet flowers, blue malva flowers, cornflowers.

purple: red and blue bases in equal parts, half as much white base (or less), santal, cinnamon, violet flowers.

white: aloes, amber, cucumber seeds, white sandalwood, camphor.

You can also add dry tempura paint powders to wood base. The amount will vary according to how much base you start out with and how deep a color you want. The colors you can achieve in this way are endless, varying from light violet to chartreuse and golden orange.

Cure your recipes in an airtight jar for a week, stirring every day until the oils are evenly absorbed. Formulate active incenses during the waxing moon, and passive incenses or incenses for Countermagic and protection during the third phase. Refrain from making incense at all during the last quarter. Use that time to clean up your work place, check which ingredients you need to reorder or gather, and think up new recipes.

Cones, Pastilles, and Sticks

Occasionally you may prefer to burn pastilles, sticks or cones instead of powdered incense. Manufacturing them is a tedious, messy process, but if you are a true "punk" enthusiast the results can be rewarding. To make them, dissolve 1 teaspoon of tragacanth gum in about 3/4 cup of water and stir until it makes a sticky paste. Add 1 ounce of saltpeter, 2 ounces of powdered charcoal, and 1/2 ounce of benzoin, myrrh, storax, or frankincense powder, musk crystals, powdered cascarilla sagrada bark, aloes, or other powdered herbs, and ten to twenty drops of fragrance.

Fold the mixture into a shallow pan and score it into pastilles. Dry them in the sun, in a 200 degree Fahrenheit oven, or for several minutes on low temperature in a microwave. When the mixture is dried, break the cones along the lines you scored, wrap them in foil, and place them in a shallow box.

If you would rather make sticks, spread the sticky mixture on broom straws and hang them upside-down from a clothes line to dry. The Chinese refined the art of joss-stick making to such a degree that they were able to tell time accurately by how long it took to burn a stick.

Never use incense-making equipment for food preparation. Make sure you thoroughly clean all bowls, measuring spoons, cups, and other equipment each time you use them, or the fragrance of one incense will mingle with the next. Keep all ingredients and equipment out of the reach of children and pets.

Planetary Incenses

Ceremonial Magicians have always set great store by burning incenses composed of ingredients ruled by the planets, which in turn, govern each day of the week, in order to draw the influence of the planet into their lives to help them be at harmony with the planetary tides and to achieve the goals which lie within the planet's rulership. Here are some planetary formulas, and the occasions and days on which to burn them during your meditations and spellwork. For more information on the planets, see *Secrets of a Witch's Coven.*

Saturn

Saturday. Rituals involving responsibilities, academic examinations, real estate, protection of the home, time, business, job performance, agriculture, compelling.

Saturn Incense

1/4 cup myrrh granules, 2 tsp. dittany of Crete, 1 tsp. crushed juniper berries, 1 Tbs. pine needles, 1 tsp. crushed ash leaves, 2 tsp. narcissus oil, 1 tsp. myrrh oil, 3/4 cup black base, 1/4 cup brown base.

Jupiter

Thursday. Rituals involving commerce, investments, banking, the law, religious or spiritual pursuits, honors, fast luck, friends, social occasions, treatises, marriages, honors, human affairs, ceremonies, peace of mind.

Jupiter Incense

1/2 cup cedar granules, 1 tsp. coumarin crystals, 1 tsp. sage, pinch of balm melissa, 1/2 tsp. nutmeg, 1/4 cup myrrh siftings, 1 tsp. carnation oil, 1/2 tsp. blue lilac oil, 1/4 tsp. clover oil, 1/2 tsp. oakmoss oil, 1/4 tsp. nutmeg oil, 1/2 tsp. clove oil, 2 tsp. amber oil, 1/2 cup blue base, 1/2 cup white base.

Mars

Tuesday. Rituals involving energy, sexuality, courage, determination, military action, enmity, protection.

Mars Incense

1 Tbs. black Indian tobacco, 1 Tbs. dragon's blood powder, 1 tsp. broom tops, 1 tsp. crushed geranium flowers, 1/2 cup frankincense peas, 1 tsp. Scotch broom oil, 1 tsp. honeysuckle oil, 1 tsp. pine oil, 1 cup red base.

Sun

Sunday. Rituals involving health, leadership, self-confidence, fame, money, good fortune, harmony, hope, friendship.

Sun Incense

1/2 cup frankincense powder, 1 tsp. saffron powder (may substitute marigold flowers or safflower petals), 1 tsp. crushed chamomile flowers, 2 tsp. cut galangal root, 1 tsp. acacia flowers, 2 tsp. heliotrope oil, 1 tsp. olibanum oil, 1 tsp. bayberry oil, 1/2 tsp. eugenol oil or cinnamon oil, 1 cup yellow base.

Mercury

Wednesday. Rituals involving commerce, communication, eloquence, performance, theft, health, influence, hidden treasures, quarrels, male fertility, spirit communications.

Mercury Incense

2 Tbs. mastic, 1/4 cup santal chips, 1/4 cup santal powder, 1 Tbs. lavender flowers, 1 tsp. cinnamon granules, 2 tsp. crushed orange peel, 2 tsp. mysore sandalwood oil, 1 tsp. neroli oil, 1/4 tsp. balm melissa oil, 1 cup orange base.

Venus

Friday. Rituals involving friendship, love, beauty, aesthetics, sex, joy, creativity, pleasure.

Venus Incense

2 Tbs. benzoin powder, 1 Tbs. white sandalwood powder, 1 tsp. angelica, 1 tsp. violet leaves, 1 Tbs. musk crystals, 1 Tbs. rose crystals, 1 tsp. vanillin, 1 tsp. white rose oil, 1/2 tsp. vanilla oil, 1 tsp. light musk oil, 3/4 cup green base, 1/4 cup white base.

Moon

Monday. Rituals involving clairvoyance, travel, fascination, spirit communication, recovery of stolen property, children, female fertility, astral travel, domestic issues, weather.

Moon Incense

1/4 cup benzoin, 1/4 cup copal resin, 1/2 tsp. camphor, 1 tsp. Irish moss, 1 tsp. jasmine flowers, 1/2 tsp. heather flowers, 1 Tbs. musk crystals, 2 tsp. cut myrtle bark, pinch of mugwort, 2 tsp. jasmine oil, 1 tsp. lotus oil, 1 tsp. magnolia oil, 1 cup white base.

Neptune

Monday. Rituals involving passion of the soul, scrying, seances, music, the subconscious mind.

Neptune Incense

1/2 cup oakmoss, 1 Tbs. crushed lotus pieces, 1 tsp. rue, 1 tsp. lotus oil, 2 tsp. dark musk oil, 1/2 tsp. opopanax oil, 1/3 cup blue base, 1/3 cup green base, 1/3 cup white base.

Uranus

Saturday. Rituals involving inventions, research, mental effort, advancement, the unusual.

Uranus Incense

1/2 cup frankincense peas, 1 Tbs. honeysuckle flowers, 1/2 tsp. galbanum oil, 1/2 tsp. coconut oil, 2 tsp. frankincense oil, 1 tsp. ambergris oil, 1 cup blue base.

Pluto

Rituals involving upheaval, the soul, the masses.

Pluto Incense

1/2 cup myrrh powder, 1/2 tsp. black powder, 1 Tbs. dragon's blood powder, 1 tsp. stephanotis oil, 1 tsp. wild rose oil, 1 tsp. copaiba oil, 3/4 cup red base, 1/4 cup black base.

Incense Formulas

Here are some formulas from my personal Book of Shadows that will give you an idea of the variety and amount of ingredients to use in your blends.

Bayberry Incense

For spells to increase prosperity, sell real estate or cars, bring business, or for the Winter Solstice:

1/2 cup frankincense siftings, 1/4 cup bayberry bark, 2 Tbs. myrrh granules, 1 Tbs. crushed bay leaves, 1 Tbs. bayberry oil, 1/2 tsp. cinnamon oil, 1 cup green base.

Damballah Incense
Calls upon the power and beneficence of the great god of the Voodoo pantheon:
1/2 cup deers tongue leaves, 2 Tbs. crushed tonka beans, 1 Tbs. cherry pipe tobacco, 1 tsp. mandrake root, 1 tsp. coumarin crystals, 1 Tbs. rum, 2 tsp. vanilla oil, 1 cup black base.

Fire-of-Love Incense
For love passionate and strong:
1 Tbs. musk ambrette crystals, 1/4 cup santal powder, 1 tsp. cinnamon granules, 1/4 tsp. allspice powder, 1 tsp. rose oil, 1 tsp. musk oil, 1/2 tsp. eugenol oil, 1/2 tsp. ylang-ylang oil, 1 cup orange base.

Gateway Incense
For those who devote their lives to the path of magical self-development; it draws the ineffable spiritual power of the All-One, and increases astral perception:
1/2 cup myrrh powder, 1 Tbs. evergreen needles, 1 tsp. honeysuckle flowers, 1 tsp. apple pieces, 1 tsp. clove powder, 1 tsp. chamomile flowers, 2 tsp. heliotrope oil, 1/2 tsp. honeysuckle oil, 1 tsp. blue sonata oil, 1/2 tsp. civet oil, 1/2 tsp. apple blossom oil, 1 tsp. spruce oil, 2 tsp. myrrh oil, 1 cup gold base.

Green Goddess Incense
A tribute to the shimmering lady of field, forest, wood, and meadow; it invokes her all-encompassing love and compassion:
1/2 cup benzoin powder, 1 tsp. rose petals, 1 tsp. heather flowers, 2 tsp. life everlasting, 1/4 cup sandalwood pieces, 1 Tbs. lemongrass, 2 tsp. vetivert, 1 tsp. rose oil, 1 tsp. wildflower oil, 1 tsp. light musk oil, 2 tsp. daisy oil, 1/2 tsp. daphne oil, 1 tsp. vetivert oil, 1/2 cup green base, 1/2 cup white base.

Heart's Desire Incense (also Libra)
To achieve your most secret wish:
1/4 cup benzoin, 1 Tbs. coumarin crystals, 2 tsp. strawberry leaves, 1 tsp. rose petals, 2 tsp. red geranium flowers, 1 tsp. primrose flowers, 1/2 tsp. thyme, 1/2 tsp. jasmine flowers, 1 tsp. verbena leaves, 1 tsp. violet leaves, 2 tsp. white rose oil, 1 tsp. primrose

oil, 2 tsp. jasmine oil, 1/2 tsp. strawberry oil, 2 tsp. violet oil, 1/2 cup green base, 1/2 cup white base.

High John/Joan the Conqueror Incense

For a successful outcome of very difficult situations, and for legal aid:

1/2 cup frankincense peas, 2 Tbs. fir needles, 1 bay leaf, crushed, 1 tsp. galangal, 1 Tbs. cedar powder, 2 tsp. frankincense oil, 1 tsp. fir oil, 1/2 tsp. cinnamon oil, 1 tsp. sweet almond oil in which 1 jalap root has been soaked for 30 days, 1/2 cup blue base.

Inner Temple

For meditation, and whenever you need to balance your energy:

2 Tbs. sandalwood powder, 1/2 cup frankincense siftings, 2 tsp. rose petals, 2 tsp. lavender flowers, 2 tsp. red rose oil, 2 tsp. parvati sandalwood oil. 1/4 tsp. lavender oil, 2 tsp. frankincense oil, 1/2 cup blue base, 1/4 cup white base.

Egyptian Khyphi Incense

Based on the Egyptian formula, Khyphi was offered to the Egyptian gods at dawn, noon, and dusk:

2 small package of raisins, 1 Tbs. red wine, 1/4 cup myrrh powder, 1/4 cup juniper berries, 1 tsp. calamus root, 2 tsp. orris powder, 2 tsp. galangal, 2 tsp. lemongrass, 2 tsp. broom flowers, 2 tsp. cardamom, 1/4 cup cinnamon, 1/2 cup frankincense siftings, 1 Tbs. honey, 1/4 cup mastic gum, 1 tsp. dragon's blood powder, 1/2 tsp. lotus oil, 1 tsp. cinnamon oil, 2 tsp. bergamot oil, 1/2 tsp. storax oil, 1/2 tsp. lemongrass oil, 2 tsp. broom oil.

Medicine Wheel

An American Indian formula for curing disease:

1/4 cup cedarwood granules, 1/4 cup lavender flowers, 1/4 cup incense cedar, 1/4 cup Yule tree needles (save from last year's tree), 1 Tbs. sage, 1 Tbs. crushed bay leaves, 2 Tbs. juniper needles, 2 tsp. spruce oil, 1/2 tsp. juniper oil. 1/2 tsp. basil oil, 1 tsp. bay rum oil.

Purification Incense

To dispel negativity from the environment:

1/2 cup myrrh gum, 1/4 cup frankincense peas, 1/4 cup frankincense powder, 1 Tbs. rosemary, 1 tsp. hyssop, 1 Tbs. lavender, 1 tsp. vervain, 1 Tbs. basil, 2 tsp. rose oil, 1/4 tsp. lemon verbena oil, 1/2 tsp. lavender oil, 2 tsp. myrrh oil.

Tree Elf Incense
Salutes the spirits called Dryads who inhabit the trees of the wild wood:
1/2 cup frankincense peas, 1/4 cup benzoin powder, 2 Tbs. fir needles, 1 Tbs. cedarwood powder, 1 Tbs. crushed lemongrass, 1 Tbs. lavender flowers, 1 tsp. Scotch broom oil, 2 tsp. Christmas pine oil, 1 tsp. mistletoe oil, 1 Tbs. wisteria oil, 1 tsp. Oriental musk oil, 2 tsp. neroli oil, 1 tsp. hyacinth oil, 1/3 cup red base, 1/3 cup purple base, 1/3 cup orange base.

Wings of Healing Incense
A sweetly gentle, yet lasting fragrance which works on a vibrational level to help heal the human organism; apply it liberally in the sickroom:
1/2 cup frankincense powder, 2 tsp. violet powder, 1 tsp. basil, 1 Tbs. lemon peel, 1 Tbs. rose oil, 2 tsp. heliotrope oil, 2 tsp. violet oil, 1/2 cup blue base, 1/2 cup pink base, 2 Tbs. white base.

Incense Candle Spell

As I mentioned earlier in this chapter, incense does not have to be burned on a coal in order to be used in a ritual. In the following ceremony you need only rub the candle with sweet almond oil, and roll it in the incense. Then light the candle and read the affirmation. Meditate on the subject of the affirmation for 5 - 15 minutes, then let the candle burn down.

I devised this spell for a friend who walked the Santiago de Compostela Trail in Spain. This ancient footpath begins in France, winds through the Spanish Pyrennes, and ends in the cathedral city of Santiago de Compostela. Since Medieval times, pilgrims have walked the trail, staying the nights in refuges, continuing on for 500 miles. The idea, besides expiation of sins, is a spiritual quest that can be taken by anyone who goes with the proper intent.

I gave my friend candles and little packages of incenses so she could light candles at churches along the way. Some of you many wonder why a Wicca Priestess would instruct anyone to worship in a church. I believe that spirituality takes many forms and that we are all following different paths to the same destination. Whether a person chooses to follow Catholicism, Protestantism, Judaism, Buddhism, Macumba, or Wicca, makes little difference as long as the person's aims are the highest. In this sense, we are all brothers and sisters on the path of Enlightenment.

Following are the intentions, incenses, candles and affirmations I suggested for my friend. By using the information in this and my other books you can devise your own personalized intentions.

Love

Fire-of-Love Incense
red candle
Affirmation: "As I light this candle I will see the way to one to whom I will be attracted to, and who will desire and honor me."

To Neutralize a Bad Situation

Purification Incense
White candle
Affirmation: "A block has been thrown up in my path, but I will not be stymied by it. I am ready, willing, and able to overcome all difficulties because my heart is full of courage and my soul is pure, and I possess the will power and strength to vanquish my adversaries."

Happy Home

Inner Temple Incense
blue candle
Affirmation: "This candle lights the way toward a tranquil home, and helps me find domestic peace, sharing, and caring."

Money-Draw

Bayberry Incense
mint green candle
Affirmation: "My intentions are good and pure. I am willing to work hard for my reward, and I have faith and confidence in the bounty of the Lord and Lady for the rewards that will soon be mine."

Success

High Joan/John the Conqueror Incense
purple candle
Affirmation: "As I light this candle, my mind, my body, and my spirit begin to work in harmony and strength to overcome all obstacles in my path. For I know that the success that I achieve is not just for myself, but also to the glory of the Ineffable Name."

Better Health

Wings of Healing Incense
red candle
Affirmation: "The merciful, healing hand of Raphael touches my body with a strong, healing pulsation, and I am well in body and whole in spirit."

Heart's Desire

Heart's Desire Incense
green candle
Affirmation: "With this web of light, I strengthen my resolve to renew the quest for my heart's desire. May this beacon open my path and bring forth the way to achieve my most cherished goals."

A Word About Incense and Scrying . . .

The way incense smoke blows is alleged to portend positive or negative events. If the smoke blows to the right, all is well; If to the left, all is lost. If it blows away from you, a bad situation will pass over, if it blows toward you, then good things are in store. If it blows both to the left and right, conditions are unsettled, and caution is advised.

Chapter 5:

Flower Power

While this entire book celebrates the undeniable influence of aromas in our lives, this chapter deals specifically with the power of flowers. Adherents of most religions -- and Wicca is no exception -- decorate their altars with flowers both as a resplendent tribute to the deity or deities and as a reminder of the eternal truths that these beautiful botanicals symbolize. In Wicca, we heap floral offerings on our altars and sometimes ring the Circle with symbolic blooms. We fashion wreaths of fresh, bright blossoms on Beltane, and crown our heads with them as a representation of the springtime of our lives. The fair garlands worn on that day help renew us mentally, physically, emotionally, and spiritually.

If you really want to experience floral energy in a hands-on way, I suggest you literally incorporate flowers into your being by eating them either during a ritual or as part of the post-rite feast. While some flowers are inedible or even poisonous, others prove quite tasty when consumed fresh as a garnish or in a salad. Some blossoms can even be candied with egg white and fine sugar and used to decorate cakes and pastries. As you would do with any plant, be sure to consult a trusted botanical guide about the safety of the plant before indulging. Imagine the "significant salad" you could concoct from some of the following edibles:

> nasturtium (patriotism)
> roses (love, unity, the ineffable)
> carnation (the eye of the god)
> clover (good luck)
> daylily buds (purity, sweetness)
> violets (faithfulness, omniscience)
> pansies (thoughts)
> squash blossoms (fertility)
> marigolds (secret knowledge gained from the fairies)
> borage blossoms (courage, merriment)
> lavender flowers (protection)
> honeysuckle (foreknowledge of fate)
> hibiscus (delicate beauty)
> jasmine (grace and elegance)
> lotus (eloquence, truth, mystery)

Toss in a variety of lettuces for bulk and background, and *voilà*! you'll serve up a very fortifying salad indeed.

Potpourri

One of the sunniest ways to honor flower power is to create potpourri. People have always enjoyed potpourri as a way to eliminate foul odors and make things smell agreeable and refreshing. Needless to say, the Egyptians were the first on record to collect and preserve flowers for their scent. Roses then, as now, constituted the primary ingredients. The Victorians probably used potpourri more than anyone. They stuffed it into headrests, armrests, and pillows to sweeten furniture, crammed it into their shoes and luggage, hung it from closet hangers and door knobs, and even festooned their Christmas trees with it.

In Magic, potpourri works better at creating an atmosphere conducive to performing spells or devotional exercises rather than setting Magic in motion. In this sense, potpourri is a passive, not an active tool. Appropriately colored, textured, and scented potpourris help drive away negativity and draw positive feelings that can alter consciousness in subtle ways. Heavenly potpourris also remind us of the magnificence of Mother Earth, and remind us to treat her with respect. I can think of few richer offerings on the altar or woodland shrine than a crystal bowlful of warmly radiating, personally crafted potpourri, I like to keep a full open container on my altar as an aid to meditation and psychic visioning.

What Goes into a Potpourri

While it requires some time and skill to make your own potpourri I think you will be pleased with the results. With the "aromamania" fashion fad that has assaulted the market lately, store-bought potpourri is easily obtainable, but the quality generally ranges from garish drugstore concoctions, where the flowers and barks are colored in a neon way unknown in Nature, to high-end "haute aromas" that cater to those who would purchase a superior image at distinctly elite prices. You will find that as you begin to select ingredients for your own potpourris, many of them will be free or inexpensive, and that $20 invested in raw materials will make a lot of potpourri.

The ingredients for potpourris are similar to those for incense. They include flowers, herbs, roots, fruit, spices, peels, and fixatives. Beautiful leaves are also a must. Whereas in incense-making you need to go easy on the rose petals because they smell like burning leaves when lighted, in potpourri, their light, natural fragrance and soft, dusky colors make them the most prized ingredient of all. Roses, therefore, form the basis for most potpourri. In general, flowers are chosen for color and texture over scent, and fragrance is added with perfume oils. Potpourri also takes advantage of unusual and beautiful mosses, even though these items usually leave no fragrance.

Almost any flower is acceptable as long as when it is dried it does not fade. Here are some suggestions for ingredients classified by color:

red - rose (flowers and buds), hollyhock, rosehip, geranium, hibiscus, clover tops, bee balm, pansy, bergamot, carnation, cockscomb;

pink - chapel flower, hollyhock, crown flower, rose (petals and buds), xeranthium (pale pinkish lavender), pirul berry, hibiscus pod;

orange - calendula, kesu flower, chapel flower, marigold, sarsparilla, nasturtium, orange peel, tansy, safflower;

yellow - life everlasting, tansy, primrose, lemon peel, Egyptian
chamomile, fructus spina christi, hops, mullein, statice,
sunflower, strawflower, buttercup, yarrow, pansy;

black - black malva, tonka bean, cubeb berry;

blue/purple - borage, cornflower, larkspur, blue malva, sweet
flag, pansy, strawflower, forget-me-not, delphinium;

brown - star anise, canella pod, buckeye, allspice berry,
cinnamon bark, cones (like hemlock, meridanium, bakuli,
lodgepole pine, casurina), senna pod, cedar shavings,
cinnamon stick, tilia star, bayberry bark, clove, juniper
berry, butterfly pod, cherry bark;

white - feverfew, windmill flower, job's tears (whitish-gray),
globe amaranth, ginger root, angel wings, yarrow, dried
mushroom, lemon peel, almond shell, orris root, pansy;

violet/purple - bouganvilla, xeranthium, heliotrope, statice,
foxglove, clover blossom, lavender, pansy, globe amaranth,
strawflower;

gray - job's tears, artemisia, benzoin, oakmoss, Spanish moss;

green - deer's tongue leaf, senna leaf, geranium leaf,
southernwood, bay leaf, violet leaf, kinnickinnick, sweet
basil leaf, lemongrass, siris leaf, sweet marjoram, sweet
woodruff, eucalyptus leaf, bergamot, sage, rosemary, apple
mint, orange mint, lemon balm, strawberry leaf, pinquinca
leaf, thyme, rosemary, patchouly.

For a stunning way to show off your potpourri, layer different
colors in a glass jar.

Besides the conventional ways of drying botanicals, you may
dry specimen flowers and herbs in borax, perlite aggregate
(available from building suppliers), silica gel, 3 parts fine white
sand and 1 part borax, or 10 parts cornmeal mixed with 2 parts
borax. These methods are good for the specimen botanicals you
wish to remain whole and brilliant so you can affix them to the
inside of the container or place them on top of it in order to show
off your potpourri to its best advantage. Alternatively, you may
wish to use a flower press or a heavy book. If you press the flowers
inside the pages of a weighty tome, wrap them first in waxed
paper.

Since roses are used more than any other flower in crafting
potpourri, I advise you hoard every rose petal you grow or receive,
and beg as many more as possible from friends. You can even

haunt florist shops for discarded blooms. You will use every rose petal you get. When I find myself in dire straits for ingredients in the dead of winter, I have been known to scrounge through the wastebasket at work for discarded bouquets given to employees on their birthdays.

To make potpourri you also need "spice." This basic ground blend includes equal amounts of at least 6 of the following spices administered in the amount of 2 Tbs. of blend per quart: allspice, anise, cardamom, coriander, caraway, cinnamon, ginger, clove, mace, nutmeg.

As in perfumery, a fixative is also necessary to even out and extend the life of the blend. Typical fixatives for potpourri include: angelica, balsam of Peru, balsam of Tolu, benzoin, frankincense, calamus, clary sage, labdanum, oakmoss, orris, sandalwood, storax, vanilla bean, and vetivert, usually in the amount of 2 Tbs. per quart, just like with the spice. Be sure the fixatives and spices are ground, not powdered unless you intend to make a sachet or put the potpourri in a non-glass container. Powder will stick to the sides of the jar and spoil the effect.

As to containers, collect small ones and large ones, woven baskets, large seashells, apothecary jars, Victorian mustard pots, cruets, decanters, biscuit tins, empty bath salts jars, decorative boxes—any pretty container that strikes your fancy, whether you see it in an antique shop or a dime store. Pretty cups or bowls covered with netting also make lovely containers. An inexpensive and inventive way to hold potpourri is to cut colored netting into squares, fill them with the blend, gather up the corners, and fasten with a bright ribbon. Basket-type containers lined with attractive material, lace, or doilies threaded with ribbon, or wooden boxes that lend their own scent to woodsy potpourris also make fine choices.

Harvesting and Drying Botanicals for Potpourri and Sachet

If you become enthusiastic about making your own potpourris and sachets you will probably want to collect some of your own ingredients because you will often find them more interesting than purchased materials. In fact, once you are really infected by the potpourri bug, you will probably never again take a walk in a garden, meadow, or forest without carrying along at least one paper or plastic bag "just in case." I have made my husband stop the car at the side of the road during a snowstorm so I could gather some tall, feathery grasses.

Any serious botanicals collector needs to know how to harvest and dry materials. In my chapter on wortcunning in *Secrets of a Witch's Coven*, I describe this procedure for medicinal botanicals, including where and when to gather them, and how to cut annuals and perennials. For potpourris and sachets you do not need to bother about the medicinal components of the botanicals, You are collecting them for color and texture only, and occasionally for fragrance. If you gather leaves or flowers for fragrance, do it in the morning after the dew has dried on the plant, but before 8:00 a.m. If you gather flowers for their beauty, you will want to wait until later in the day after the blooms have opened to their fullest glory. Barks, seeds, roots, resins and peels can be harvested at any time, but bark is best taken while the tree is dormant.

Bring along a flower press to capture the beauty of the best specimens while they are fresh. Small, lightweight presses are available that handily fit into a backpack.

Gather seeds when they are fully ripe, but have not yet fallen to the ground. If you are going for roots, wait until the end of the growing season, and pull up the entire plant. Cut them into small chunks 1/2" - 1" across, and place the pieces on a drying screen. Wash the leaves to remove all the dirt; throw away dead or browning leaves, strip the good ones from the stalk carefully, and dry them on a screen. Some flowers also can be dried on a screen without shrivelling; others need to be pressed.

Peel vertical strips of bark when the tree is dormant, taking care not to take so much that you damage the tree. Pin the strips on a clothes line with a wooden clothespin to dry; then chip them into pieces.

Finally, when preparing peels, scrape out the white pulp, cut into squares, and arrange the pieces on the screen to dry. Peels shrink when dried, so you need to cut the pieces about 20% larger than you want them to be when they are dry.

Use wire screens. Place the botanicals on the screen leaving space between them, and cover with a piece of cheesecloth to protect them from wind and dust. Stacked screens, like the kind used for drying fruit and vegetables, make efficient driers.

Some fragrance crafters recommend drying botanicals in a microwave or warm oven. Although this works well for medicinal herbs, the heat may shrivel or brown the plant, which ruins it for potpourri (but not necessarily for sachet). At least this has been my experience in Colorado's semi-arid climate.

As with all aspects of fragrance crafting, I advise you to label each botanical because sometimes the final results are not easy to distinguish, especially when you are drying artemisias and mints.

Potpourri-Making Methods

Two basic ways to make potpourri have been developed. The moist method is more time-consuming, and the results should be kept in a container that cannot be seen through, because the ingredients lose their color due to the bleaching action of the salt that is required to make it. The advantage of moist potpourri is that it lasts practically forever.

To make a moist potpourri, place a 1/2" layer of partially dried flower petals that have lost about 1/3 of their bulk into a crock or large pot. Follow with a 1/2" layer of non-iodized salt, or salt and brown sugar. Cover with a piece of glass, and press down with a heavy weight on the glass.

Stir the mixture with a wooden spoon each day. After about 10 days, a hard cake of scented matter will form. Remove the cake, crumble it, and set it aside with the spices and fixatives. You may add several layers of petals and salt as you obtain more partially dried ingredients. After the hard cake forms, the first step in the aging process is complete. Stir in the spices, leaves, roots, oils, fixatives, and crumbled cake. Return the mixture to the crock, and stir for 2 weeks or longer until the scent matures. The more you age the mixture, the longer it will retain its fragrance.

Some moist potpourri recipes call for bay salt. To make your own, crush 6 bay leaves in 1 pound of salt until they are exhausted.

The dry method creates a more subtly scented, brilliantly colored potpourri with a lot less fuss, but one whose fragrance needs to be reactivated from time to time by adding more oils and fixative, or a tablespoon of brandy.

Dry petals, herbs, and other ingredients using the above described methods until they are the consistency of cornflakes. Place the materials in a pot with a tight lid and add 2 Tbs. of spice and 2 Tbs. of fixative per quart of petals. Add up to 1 Tbs. of the oils you wish to use (1 Tbs. all together). Mix well, and close the lid tightly. Stir the mixture every day for about 6 weeks, checking the scent each week to see if it needs more spice or oil. After about 6 weeks when the mixture has matured, remove it and spoon it loosely into a clear container. Attach especially striking flower specimens to the inside of the container with egg white before filling. Egg white will not leave an ugly yellow mark on the side of the glass like glue often does. Crown the container with some of your prettiest flowers, cones and berries. If you have an open container, cover it with netting so that the fragrance can escape while the flowers stay snugly in place.

Sachets

In an earlier chapter you learned to make simple sachets to scent letters in order to subliminally communicate secret desires. Now that you know how to make potpourri, you can concoct more sophisticated sachets. Sachets are simply potpourri that has been aged for three weeks or more, and ground to a powder. Because ground botanicals release their fragrance quickly, at least 50% of the sachet should be a fixative, which is a higher percentage than required for potpourri. If you need to increase the bulk, add wood base, cornstarch, or arrowroot starch, all of which readily absorb the oils.

For a standard drawer, closet, or purse sachet, the easiest, and one of the prettiest containers I've found is an embroidered hanky. Place sachet powder in the middle, and tie the corners of the hanky together with a colorful ribbon. To renew your sachet's fragrance without staining the cloth, dab some perfume or essential oil on a cotton ball, open the hanky, and nestle the cotton into the powder. Be sure the fabric you choose is closely woven so that the ingredients cannot escape.

Here are some sachet recipes:

Moth-Away

2 parts each of cedarwood, sassafras, vetivert; 1 part each of bay leaf, rosemary, tansy, southernwood; 1/2 part each of camphor and wormwood. Enhance this blend with essential oil of any of the above ingredients.

Flea Fly Away

Equal parts chamomile, pennyroyal, and rue. Round out the blend with essential oils.

Fly Fly Away
Equal parts cedarwood, sandalwood, and vetivert, plus some citronella oil.

Graveyard Dust
Used in Voodoo to cross a person. Usually the practitioner dusts the doorway or threshold where the enemy will cross.
1 oz. mullein; 1 oz. wormwood; 13 patchouly leaves, crushed; 1 oz. alder leaves; crushed, 1 oz. bone ash (you may substitute black or a mixture of black and white and brown incense base); 1 oz. mandrake, crushed.

House Protection Sachet
To hang over the inside of the door or window, or to place in the corner of a room.
equal parts basil, periwinkle, cedar powder, rosemary powder, elder flowers.

Binding Powder
To bind spells
1 part incense coal, crushed; 2 parts frankincense powder; 2 parts myrrh powder; 1 oz. santal powder; 1 ounce black coral, crushed, "magnetic filings," vesta powder.

Powders in Magic

Sachet-type powders have been used in Magic for centuries. Time after time the Old English Herbals warned against "elf-shot," a deadly powder that was thought to cause infectious diseases. The way to counteract the deadly venom, so it was believed, was to concoct a sachet of powdered mugwort, plantain, chamomile, nettles, crabapple, chervil, and fennel.

Modern Witches still use powders in rituals and spellcasting in an intriguing variety of ways. A package can be placed inside a Voodoo poppet, under a pillow, inside a mailbox, beneath the bed sheets, inside an envelope and mailed, or inside a lingerie drawer. Powders can be sprinkled in Circle during a spell, added directly to sigils and perfumes, used as a dressing for candles, scattered at the entrance to a house or room, placed at the bottom of an incense burner, burned as incense, rubbed on the wrists, temples, waist, feet, and ankles, layered on an open book page, placed in a potpourri jar, dispersed around the altar, or blown to the Four Quarters.

Typical Witches' powder ingredients include the following:

asoefetida - returns psychic attacks to the perpetrator

basil - entices customers to a store

brimstone - foils enemies

camphor - attracts the power of the moon

cayenne - makes things happen; brings quick action

cinnamon - attracts excitement and adventure

clove - dissolves discord

frankincense - dispels bad dreams

grains of paradise - draws love

lavender - attracts good luck

mustard - aids against psychic attack

nutmeg - activates a love spell

pepper - banishes despair; rids one of enemies

rosebud - a love spell powder

rosemary - protects in travel

sandalwood - heals; binds spells

salt - confers blessings

vanilla - brings good fortune.

These powders are usually mixed in a base of cornstarch and baking soda.

Spell of the Seven Powders

I wish to share with you a very special ritual that I once created for our coven. It seems that many people I know in the Craft do not believe that we should ever perform any spellwork for ourselves, for our own gain. They point to the fates of many erstwhile Magicians who let themselves become so enamored with cosmic power that they twisted it to suit their own ends, thereby bringing about their own destruction.

It is true that as human beings we need to be aware of our failings and strive not to get carried away by the Light that surges through us. Yet at the same time, if we let ourselves fall into ill health or be so consumed with trying to eke out a living that we cannot think of anything but our own survival, what good are we as healers? We need to be strong and well-balanced as part of becoming ideal vehicles through which to move the Cosmic Light.

If this means that we occasionally need to perform spellwork to ease our worldly burdens, then there is no harm in it, as long as we harm no one else. We put ourselves into a better position to continue with the Great Work. Not abuse, but judicious, moderate, occasional use of this power is as it should be.

With these words of advice, I introduce you to the Spell of the Seven Powders, the aim of which is to bring a little needed prosperity into your life.

This ceremony is designed specifically to draw money to the participants. It is not appropriate to wish for success, good luck, fruition of plans, etc. in a general manner. By narrowing the focus, the participants are more likely to achieve their aims.

As a ritual for wealth and increase, we draw upon the powers of Jupiter. Jupiter is the energy that governs riches, employment, trade, honors, and hope. Translated into symbolic form, he is the jovial god; so create an atmosphere in the Circle of openness, friendliness, self-confidence, and happiness. From the moment the participants begin to arrive, play an appropriately upbeat tape or record in the background to help establish this carefree mood.

We partake of food and drink during the ritual, in part, to promote sociability. Creme de mènthe is drunk because of its association with mint (a money-drawing herb) and because of its color, which is also the color of money and prosperity. Cut the "Sugar Daddy Cookies" in the form of an egg, the symbol of creativity and fertility, in order to carry through the analogy of increase.

The unicorn, which plays a part in the ritual, is a symbol of Jupiter, along with the blue carnations and figs for the altar. All the botanicals and perfumes either are directly related to Jupiter, and/or to prosperity and money.

Items Required

Seven Sachet Powders
To prepare these powders, unless otherwise directed, grind 1 tablespoonful of each botanical to a powder with a mortar and pestle. Mix all the powders botanicals together. Add four drops of each indicated perfume oil ("four" is the number of Jupiter), and stir the mixture. Store in airtight containers.

"Circle Purification Powder" - to purify and consecrate the Circle; 2 parts sandalwood, 1 part violet flowers, 1 part rose petals, 1/2 part hyssop, 1 oak leaf, Oriental oil, violet oil.

"Treasure Powder" - to sprinkle on the altar and rub on the altar candles; 1 ounce almond flour, 8 drops bitter almond oil.

"Jupiter Powder" - to rub on the petition candles and to add to the incense; 3 parts cedar, 1 part rose, 8 drops rose oil, 4 drops cedar oil, 4 drops jasmine oil.

"Invocation Powder" - to blow toward each Quarter when invoking the Archangels; equal parts frankincense and myrrh, no oils.

"Dagda Powder" - to charge the magical seals; 4 parts myrrh, 2 parts fir needles, 1 part anise seed, pine oil, sage oil, civet oil, 1 drop peppermint oil.

"Gypsy Gold Powder" - to charge the charm bags; equal parts cinnamon, nutmeg, mistletoe, carnation, carnation oil, rose oil, 1 drop patchouly oil.

"Wealthy Way Powder" - to take home to sprinkle in the corners of each room, on the threshold, or to carry to your place of business, and rub on the cash register and doorknob; equal parts cinnamon, frankincense, chamomile, calendula, basil, 1 bay leaf; 4 drops each almond oil, frankincense oil, bayberry oil, 2 drops patchouly oil.

2 blue carnations in a vase for the altar.

A small bowlful of figs as an offering—these may be canned.

The tarot card, Wheel of Fortune, for meditation.

1 green or brown candle for each petitioner; candle holders.

Parchment, scissors, and a blue pen to make the seals.

Sky-blue Jupiter altar candles.

Jupiter-blue altar cloth.

Green, 2"-square charm bag with drawstring for each petitioner.

Unicorn symbol painted on a piece of tin (figure 5.1). This could be as simple as a picture on a piece of tin foil wrapped around a square of cardboard. If you cannot find an appropriate piece of tin, and you have a unicorn necklace, ring, or earring, this will do.

Herbs for charm bags: basil, cinnamon, cinquefoil, clover, and almond and peppermint oils.

Jupiter incense, incense burner, quick-lighting coal, matches.

Small bottle of crème de menthe, cordial glasses for petitioners. Do not drink from the Sacred Cup.

Sugar Daddy Cookies:

2 sticks softened butter
1 cup sugar
1 egg
2 teaspoons baking powder
1 teaspoon almond extract
1 teaspoon vanilla extract
2-1/4 cups unsifted flour

Combine butter, sugar, the extracts, egg, baking powder and flour. Cover and chill for 2 hours. Roll out 1/8" thick on a floured board and cut into 2-1/2" ovoid forms. Bake at 350 F. degrees for 8 - 10 minutes. Remove cookies from oven; allow them to cool completely. Frost with tubes of green and blue frosting, writing the name of each participant on a cookie.

The Rite

On a Thursday when the moon is waxing, but not yet full, erect an altar in the West. Cover it with the Jupiter altar cloth, and place the two altar candles on either side at the back. Between the candles, place the vase of carnations, and in front of it, the bowl of figs. Prop up the tarot card in front of the bowl of figs for the participants to contemplate as the ritual unfolds. Place the incense burner at the front left side of the altar, and the unicorn symbol at the front right side. Lay your Athame and Invoking Rod across the front center of the altar. Position the crème de menthe, cordial glasses, and Pentacle heaped with cookies in front of the altar.

Opening the Circle

Participants take their places, sitting around the Circle, quietly meditating on the Wheel of Fortune and their material needs. The same participant should prepare the Circle Purification Powder and Treasure Powder. This participant begins the rite by ringing the Circle with Purification Powder, and sprinkling the altar with Treasure Powder.

The person who prepared the Jupiter Powder rubs it on the altar candles, lights the coal, sprinkles on the incense, and adds some Jupiter Powder to the incense.

The Priestess opens the Circle with the Lesser Banishing and Invoking Pentagram Rituals. At each Quarter, as she finishes the invoking segment of the ritual, she takes up the Invocation Powder, and blows it toward the Quarter.

Priestess: "The purpose of this ritual is to attract money and wealth to each and every member of our group. It is not often that we use our Wise Ways to draw material benefits. Yet there comes a time when we cannot continue to help others, increase our own self-awareness, nor pursue higher knowledge for the good of all unless our physical needs are met on this earthly plane. Spiritual development is more readily attained when we are not forced to depend on others who might seek to control and manipulate us through our basic needs.

"We do not ask for excessive amounts of money, nor certainly for anything at the expense of others. However, as Western Witches and Magicians, we live in the real world, which requires money as a means of exchange for goods and services. Moreover, if we cannot demonstrate that we can perform Magic successfully for ourselves, how can we be expected to do so for others?

"With these considerations in mind, we now invoke Dagda, the All-Father of the Irish fairies, who in other traditions is known as Amon, Poseidon, Thor, and Zeus. We call upon Dagda to aid us in our Magic, and to offer us his brimming Cornucopia-Cauldron, from which no petitioner goes away unsated."

Invocation of Dagda

Priest:
"Dagda, father of the Tuatha de Dannan,
Dagda of the Magic Club,
Dagda, the All-Father,
Dagda of the Cornucopia-Cauldron
Dagda, who rejects no one,
Dagda, Lord of Perfect Knowledge,
We call upon you, Dagda, Dagda, Dagda!
Join us here and now, Dagda, Dagda, Dagda,
Come to our Circle of Light,
Come, and nourish your needy people!"
All:
"Dagda! Dagda! Dagda! "

Rite of the Unicorn

The guardian of the Jupiter Powder now distributes it to the participants to rub on their candles. Begin at the bottom of the candle, and rub the powder in a continuous circular motion toward the center. Begin again at the top, and rub to the center.

The Priestess lights her petition candle and places it on the altar, then takes the unicorn symbol in her hands, and while holding it, tells Dagda and the participants how much money she expects to obtain from the spell, and why. She passes the unicorn deosil around the Circle, and each participant follows her example by lighting a petition candle, and declaring a desire. When the unicorn is returned to the Priestess, she places it back on the altar. In this way, everybody has a clear idea of what is required, and can concentrate on these goals during the seal charging rite.

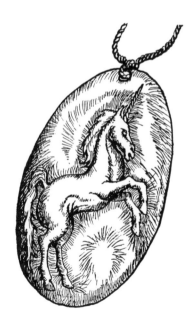

Figure 5.1

Unicorn Painted on Tin in Blue or White

Rite of the Sacred Seal

Next, the guardian of the charm bags and herbs distributes them, and the participants fill their pouches, leaving room for the seals. They add apinch of Gypsy Gold Powder to the herbs in the bags, hold the bags closed, and shake well to evenly distribute the powder. They they each cut a circle from the parchment small enough to fit inside the bag, and draw the seal with the blue pen. The seal consists of the Kamea (Square) of Jupiter (figure 5.2) on one side, with the petitioner's first name reduced to numbers drawn on it (to find out how to reduce names to numbers, see figure 5.4). On the other side, the petitioners trace the Qabalistic signatures of the planet's angelic forms (figure 5.3).

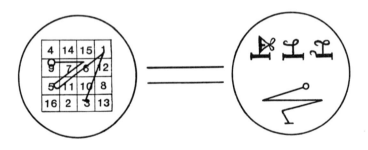

Figure 5.2	Figure 5.3
Kamea of Jupiter with the name "Rowan" drawn on it in numbers.	Sachiel: Archangel of Jupiter Iophiel: Intelligence of Jupiter

Archangel : Sachiel

Intelligence: Iophiel

They anoint their seals with cinnamon oil on one side, and clover oil on the other side, tracing with their fingers dipped in the oils, an unbroken circle around the perimeter of the seal on each side. Place one drop of almond oil in the center of each side. Then they sprinkle Dagda Powder on top of the seals.

When finished, the participants place their seals with the numbers side up on top of the charm bags, and lay them in the middle of the circle. The group joins hands and chants:

Figure 5.4
Table for Reducing Numbers

1	2	3	4	5	6	7	8	9
A	B	C	D	E	F	G	H	I
J	K	L	M	N	O	P	Q	R
S	T	U	V	W	X	Y	Z	
R = 9		O = 6		W = 5		A = 1		N = 5

All: "O Mane Padme Hum"

When the chant has raised a cone of power and reaches its climax, they drop hands, and direct the energy raised by the cone toward the charms, focusing on everybody's wishes.

Rite of Cakes and Ale

The Priest pours the crème de menthe into the cordial glasses, blesses the liqueur and the cookies, and distributes them to the participants. Everybody eats, drinks, and makes merry, chatting about their plans of what they will do with their newly-acquired wealth.

Closing the Circle

When the time is appropriate, the Priestess rises and faces the altar. The participants quiet down, and she says,

Priestess: "Within the Celtic magical system nine laws exist that have been given to us by the Muses of the Sacred Cauldron. The ninth of these commandments is called The Law of Abundance. It states that `like attracts like.' In other words, money attracts money, and fear of poverty is actually an unrequited wish. I leave you with this thought as you exchange this Circle of Light for the glow of the other world: in order to obtain money you must spend some money, and it is best spent for a good cause. Spend more, and riches will be returned to you."

The Priestess performs the Banishing Pentagram Ritual to close the Circle. The participants leave with their candles and baggies of Wealthy Way Powder to use at their own discretion. For example, at the next full moon, a petitioner might sprinkle some on the candle, and burn it down, while meditating on ways to increase wealth. Money and riches are now coming your way!

Chapter 6:

Heaven-Scents to Heal Body, Mind and Spirit

So far this book has been concerned with the psychological effects of scents and how they can be used to create changes in consciousness. This branch of healing attracts many Witches because it combines our knowledge of Magic with the commitment to help others. The physical side of healing is often left to the physician trained in Medicine.

Time was when Witchcraft and Medicine enjoyed a closer relationship. In the days when surgeons were considered nothing better than glorified barbers and had not yet designed and developed a theoretical framework, coherent body of knowledge, or course of rigorous study, the village wise woman or wise man was the healer the people visited in times of illness, stress, or any deviation from behavioral norms. This highly respected community member, often a Witch, possessed vast, empirically proven knowledge of botanicals, and could be depended on to alleviate many ailments.

As the medical profession developed, doctors needed to do something to increase their credibility with the people. Logically, to them, this meant discrediting the herbal healers bringing them down so the doctors could step into their shoes. According to

Mary Chamberlain in *Old Wives Tales*, doctors closed ranks and did not let anyone study new advances in medicine with them who had not been recommended by one of their number, and who could not afford the tuition. This left the Witch healers out of the money. Then, aided and abetted by the Church and State, who had their own reasons for believing Witches were dangerous, the medical and official establishment mounted a defamation campaign against the herbalists. Since they could not compete with new discoveries in the health field, and because they were persecuted by the powers who saw their popularity with the people as a threat, Witches and other healers were eventually driven underground.

> One can ... see why physicians and surgeon/apothecaries were united in their opposition to old wives. In the making of this professional caste, the doctors were prepared to sink their intra-professional jealousies to defeat a rival tradition and practice.

> What is unique about this situation is the scale of the struggle it represented. For the attempt to eradicate the old wife's practice was not simply a question of the evolution of knowledge within a discipline...It was a move to outlaw a body of knowledge and its practitioners, involving the total defeat of a tradition which stood as a direct antithesis to it.[8]

Only at the end of the twentieth century, have those now called "alternative healers" been able to recuperate any semblance of the dignity and authority they once enjoyed. All ideas seem to pass through cycles, and notions about health are no exception. Modern Medicine has prevailed now for several centuries, and as with probably any organization, it has in some ways grown complacent, unwilling to make changes in established routines. This attitude simply reflects human nature in that we all tend to resist change. The fresh, sometimes revolutionary approaches put forth by some New Age healers often are condemned out-of-hand as bizarre, silly, or even dangerous to human health. Certainly, charlatans and well-meaning "inepts" (as opposed to "adepts") exist in any field, including all branches of Medicine. And it is not my purpose in writing this book to defend every nook and cranny of the New Age movement.

Yet as I see the medical profession growing more resistant to change I believe that many alternative healing theories are just what the doctor ordered to inject vitality back into health care.

Many of these techniques seem to fill spaces where traditional Medicine apparently has not worked. Ironically, the New Age healers often use age-old methods which, with a contemporary twist, harken back to the times of the Witch healers. Here is where aromatherapy fits into the Witch's healing pouch, and why I address it with a chapter in this book.

Another reason to talk about aromatherapy is that it has become a buzz word in the alternative healing community which has spread out and infected the general population. Because most people do not take the time to understand the theories, all sorts of misconceptions have arisen as to the panaceian powers of aromatherapy to cure every malaise under the sun. As usual, the truth lies somewhere in between.

Aromatherapy is the technique by which essential oils are ingested, applied externally to the skin, or inhaled in order to heal the body, emotions, mind, and spirit. Essential oils have been defined elsewhere in this book (see chapter 2), but it is useful to note that these highly volatile, concentrated vegetable substances possess a complex chemical organization that integrates well with the human organism. As Jean Valnet in *The Practice of Aromatherapy* points out, "essences present more new compounds than the chemists of the whole world could analyze in a thousand years...they are mixtures of many constituents: terpenes, alcohols, esters, aldehydes, ketones, and phenols, etc." [9]

The Pros and Cons of Aromatherapy

Before extolling the virtues of essential oils in aromatherapy, it is probably a good idea to note their drawbacks.

In the above quotation Valnet himself refers to terpenes as one of the constituents of essences. Terpenes can be harmful to humans and animals, and especially can irritate the skin. They can be "cleaned" from essential oils, but then this raises the question of whether the oil rendered is really natural. Some essential oils like thuja, which is derived from the *Arbor vitae* tree native to China and North America, are poisonous and cannot be ingested.

So all essential oils are not necessarily safe for the body.

Since true essences are distilled naturally from botanicals, it takes a lot of plant matter, and much labor intensive work to produce enough saleable oil. These days, with people clamoring for natural fragrances coupled with the worldwide rising costs of labor, few essential oils can be harvested and distilled at a price affordable to anyone. Because the oils are so expensive, many are adulterated with synthetic esters, alcohol, and essences of lesser value, so you need to find an honest manufacturer if you plan to use pure essences. Moreover, it takes many essential oils a long time to work on the body because they cause subtle changes. If a patient is in a bad way, the essential oil may work too slowly to be effective.

On the other hand, many essential oils possess the physiochemical ability to prevent putrification, destroy bacteria, lessen inflammation, and with their high concentration of hormones and vitamins, defend the body against disease and serve as a tonic.

They also create a synergistic effect in that they combine with the body's chemistry in such a way that the impact of the whole is greater than the sum of its parts. Essences are especially adept at bringing about a balance of body, mind, and emotion -- attributes that are almost unknown in pharmaceutical medications.

As you have learned in earlier chapters, scent goes directly to the limbic system and can stimulate emotional as well as physical behavior. It is no accident that oils are associated with cosmetics, because the Greek root of the word "cosmetic" is *kosmea*, which means "to harmonize."

Some essential oils which act as strong bactericides include clove, verbena, lavender, patchouly, angelica, juniper, sandalwood, cedar, thyme, lemon, pine, wormwood, jasmine, tuberose, anise, and valerian. For example, essence of lavender and eucalyptus will kill the typhoid bacillus in 45 minutes and tuberculosis in 12 hours.[9]

Hardly a day goes by without some new miracle cure attributed to botanicals popping into the news. For example, Linda Fellows, biochemist at Kew Gardens, England, discovered that an extract from the seeds of the *Castanospermum australe*, an Australian rain forest tree, appears to have a strong blocking effect on the HIV virus as well as being an insecticide, at least in the laboratory.

The extract is now undergoing testing in the U.S., where the substance is known as Oxald.[10] Such news is exciting for more than the eradication of AIDS. It provides proof that curing disease with botanicals is a viable alternative for the 4 billion people on the planet from underdeveloped nations who must rely on herbs as an inexpensive alternative to pharmaceutical medicines.

You may wonder why the drug companies have not snatched up the gauntlet and intensively combed the botanical storehouse for raw material to create new drugs. Stephen Foster in an article for *Harrowsmith* [11] tells us that currently it costs $100 - 125 million to provide test data to the FDA to deem a product safe for human consumption. Coupled with the notable lack of public funding for such research and the fact that the company doing the testing will not necessarily end up with exclusive rights to market the product, botanical drug testing becomes a decidedly unattractive corporate pursuit.

With the recent attempt on the part of the government combined with the power of the pharmaceutical industries and the medical profession to crack down on distribution of vitamins, herbs, and aromatherapeutic products, the people's right to take care of themselves is being threatened. Still, we can only hope that the American values of individual freedom and self-reliance will prevail and we will be allowed to self-medicate unimpeded by government interference. This is one of the reasons why this chapter and the book itself are being written: to help people understand the principles of aromatherapy and what the technique can do to help people become and stay healthy.

Historical Capsule

Healing with aromatics is not a new concept. Ayurvedic Medicine, which has always used essential oils as part of its medicine chest, has been in continuous practice in India for 10,000 years.

The Chinese pharmacopeia of 2,000 years ago the *Pen Tsao*, whose authorship is attributed to the emperor Shen Nung, records some remedies comprised of essences. Ancient people around the globe, like the Egyptians, Hebrews, Anglo-Saxons, and American Indians believed in "smoking" or fumigating patients with herbs from fires and smudge sticks to alleviate pain and cure disease. The Egyptians, for example, heated up large vessels filled with botanicals and water. Over the opening they placed a piece of wool cloth that would become impregnated with the essential oil as the steam arose from the pot. They wrung out the oil from the cloth, and took it internally.

You have already learned that the Arabs were the first to distill essences with alcohol. The Renaissance Alchemists in their spiritual quest for the elixir of life, refined these distillation techniques by inventing the refrigerated coil, and evolved more and stronger methods of extraction. Before the advent of modern chemistry and the drugs this science produced, the Alchemists' essences formed the basis of most medicinal treatments.

With the birth of the modern pharmaceutical industry, healing with essential oils fell out of the picture, that is, until the twentieth century, when it experienced a revival. As the French rank as undisputed leaders in the perfume industry, so they are also the great innovators in the field of aromatherapy. In fact, the French chemist, Rene-Maurice Gattefossé coined the term "aromatherapy" in a book he published on the subject in 1937, which earned him the title Father of Aromatherapy. His work was expanded by Fesneau, Caujolles, and Pellecuer.

Another Frenchman, Dr. Jean Valnet, used his predecessors' techniques to treat soldiers injured in World War II. Valnet had several students, one of whom, Marguerite Maury, transported his theories across the Channel to England, and hence to the English-speaking world. At the same time, Valnet awakened interest in Germany, Switzerland and Italy, notably in Milan, where research has been done, for example, into the treatment with aromatherapy of hysteria and depression.

An offshoot of aromatherapy which depends on flowers for healing was developed by Dr. Bach, who floated flowers in spring water and kept them in the sun to let the water become impregnated with solar and floral energy. His remedies for pain, intolerance, life transitions, exhaustion, etc., have become world-renowned.

How to Administer Essential Oils

Essential oils are used in three ways: inhalation, external application to the body, and internal ingestion. Previous chapters have dealt with inhalation in incenses, sachets, and potpourris.

External application can be in a bath and facial saunas (which also include an element of inhalation), and frictions, lotions, liniments, and massage oils as well as occasionally enemas or douches. It takes about a half hour to two hours for external applications to the skin to be completely absorbed by the body.

For the best absorption of a friction it is a good idea to warm the skin. Afterwards, cover the affected area with a damp compress for even more effective penetration.

Essential oils are usually taken internally to aid digestive problems and help cure infections. They can be ingested as is, or diluted in 80% ethyl alcohol, sweet almond oil, olive oil or vinegar, or mixed with water, honey, in drops on a sugar cube, or added to other medicines.

I suggest that you never take essential oils externally or internally without the guidance of a trained aromatherapist or doctor. Some essences, even in minute amounts, can be extremely dangerous. Also, aromatherapeutic and homeopathic treatments are not compatible; they tend to cancel each other out.

It is not the purpose of this chapter to teach you how to prepare your own formulas for aromatherapy, but for you to increase your general knowledge in case you, or anyone you know is seeking treatment. You should familiarize yourself with some of the terms aromatherapists use, and be aware of the curative properties of some of the more popular essential oils in order to broaden your appreciation of essences in general.

Terminology

Here are some terms you should know if you intend to pursue the art of aromatherapy.

Acetum - a preparation obtained by mixing aromatic substances in vinegar.

Aroma Lamp - a small container that heats water by using a candle or a light bulb. Add a few drops of essential oil to the heated water to gently diffuse the aroma throughout the room. An aroma lamp is especially effective in the sick room or when you wish to create a subtle atmosphere.

Compound - a mixture of chopped or crushed plants which share the same curative properties, and that can be used to make decoctions and infusions.

Compress - a wet or dry folded material that is applied externally to the body.

Cordial - a sweet tonic and stimulant usually ingested to invigorate the heart. Often it is prepared with alcohol.

Decoction - a liquid preparation obtained by boiling in a covered enamel pot plant parts (usually the roots and thicker stems) in water for at least 15 minutes. The mixture will lose at least 2/3 of its water. The liquid is then strained and ingested. Since a decoction uses plant parts rather than their essences, it is not strictly considered an aromatherapeutic preparation.

Elixir - a preparation obtained from sweetened aromatics and alcohol.

Embrocation - a method of external application whereby part of the body is sprinkled with an aromatherapeutic liquid, which is then rubbed into the skin. It is also called a friction rub.

Extract - a medicinal preparation obtained by partially evaporating a tincture. An extract is about 4 to 6 times stronger than a tincture. A fluid extract, or liquid extract is made by mixing a drug with several times its weight of alcohol or water, and then evaporating the liquid until its weight equals the original weight of the drug.

Floral Water/ Aromatic Water - a preparation obtained by sending steam made from distilled water through plant material, then condensing the steam. It is also known as a hydrolate. Floral waters may be ingested, but more often are splashed on the body for skin care. Popular examples include rose, lavender, and orange waters.

Fomentation - a warm, moist preparation obtained from a liquid that is applied externally by hand, brush, cloth or sponge in order to assuage pain and reduce inflammations.

Fumigation - a preparation obtained by boiling plants in water and having the patient inhale the vapor. A facial sauna is a common type of fumigation that is used to open pores, tighten skin, clear up acne, etc.

Homeopathy - a system of healing advocating the administration of small doses of a drug that would in a healthy person produce symptoms of the disease being treated. In simplistic terms, it is something akin to "the hair of the dog that bit you." Many aromatherapists claim that homeopathy and aromatherapy treatments if applied simultaneously, cancel each other out.

Infusion - a preparation obtained by boiling the more tender parts of a plant or plants, like the flowers, leaves, and soft stems in water to extract their actual properties, then straining and ingesting the liquid. An infusion differs from a decoction in that usually the more tender parts of the plant are used, and they are boiled for less time, usually from 5 to 15 minutes. Like a decoction, an infusion is not strictly considered aromatherapeutic medicine. An infusion is more concentrated than a tea.

Lotion - a liquid preparation that is applied externally to the skin as a lubricant, astringent, cleanser, and softener.

Ointment/Balsam - an unctious preparation meant to heal and soothe wounds obtained by mixing distilled essences with a greasy base like oil or fat, and a solidifier like lanolin or beeswax. If the ointment is prepared with wax, it is called a cerate. The result is then applied externally. A plaster is like an ointment, only it is meant to adhere to the body.

Syrup - a preparation obtained by mixing sugar and an herbal preparation in cold or hot water. Syrups are usually used for coughs, sore throats, and respiratory ailments.

Tea - a tea is prepared like a decoction or infusion, but the water is only brought to a boil, then turned off to let the plant parts steep for about 5 minutes before the preparation is consumed. A tea is milder than a decoction or an infusion, and usually tastes pleasant enough to be considered a beverage. For a complete discussion of teas in healing and Magic, see my book, *Green Magic*, Whitford Press, 1993.

Tincture - a solution which is rendered by keeping fresh plant parts usually crushed or chopped in alcohol, water, or sweet almond or olive oil for several weeks in the quantity of one part plant material by weight to 5 parts liquid. The liquid is then strained and ingested. Tinctures are usually diluted with water, vinegar, wine, or honey, or sprinkled on a sugar cube.

Tisane - An infusion of flowers usually formed into a cake with sugar or honey that is then melted in hot water and consumed as a beverage. Popular tisanes include chamomile, peppermint, and rose hips. Agatha Christie's world-renowned detective, Hercule Poirot never fails to imbibe his daily tisane to ward off the cold germs engendered by the damp, frigid English climate.

Tonic - a preparation that restores and invigorates the system.

Essential Oils for 36 Common Complaints

The following list gives you an idea of some of the essences you can use to help cure physical and mental ailments.

You will need to check a book on aromatherapy such as those listed in the bibliography, or do some testing on your own to establish the correct dosages.

Acne - cajeput, juniper, lavender.

Anemia - chamomile, garlic, lemon, thyme.

Arthritis - cajeput, camphor, juniper, thyme.

Asthma - aniseed, cajeput, balm, clary, eucalyptus, rosemary, hyssop, lemon, garlic, naiouli, origanum, peppermint, pine.

Bleeding - cypress, lemon.

Cancer - clove, cypress, garlic, geranium, hyssop, onion, sage, tarragon.

Conjunctivitis - rose, chamomile, lemon.

Coughs - cypress, hyssop, fennel, aniseed, thyme, myrtle, eucalyptus.

Depression - chamomile, lavender, thyme, bergamot, balm, neroli, rose, yarrow, ylang-ylang, pine, basil, geranium, nutmeg.

Diarrhea - neroli, sandalwood, cypress, savory, cajeput, nutmeg, clover, chamomile, geranium, cinnamon, ginger, juniper, lavender, neroli, peppermint, rosemary, sage.

Digestion - angelica, lemon verbena, mint, clary, orange, tarragon, aniseed, basil, bergamot, chamomile, clove, fennel, ginger, lemongrass, juniper, lavender.

Earache - cajeput, lavender, savory.

Fatigue - basil, cinnamon, clove, eucalyptus, garlic, geranium, ginger, hyssop, lavender, lemon, marjoram, nutmeg, rosemary, thyme.

Flu - camphor, chamomile, cinnamon, cypress, eucalyptus, fennel, garlic, hyssop, lavender, lemon, niaouli, onion, peppermint, pine, rosemary, sage, thyme.

Headache - lavender, balm, neroli, ginger, chamomile, marjoram, rose, lemon, clary, basil, ylang-ylang, peppermint, yarrow.

Hemorrhoids - myrtle, garlic, cypress, onion, yarrow.

Hiccups - basil, dill, fennel, tarragon.

Insect Bites - lavender, basil, balm, cinnamon, mint, sage, lemon, thyme, tea tree.

Insomnia - neroli, marjoram, rosewood, sandalwood, rose, lavender.

Kidneys - eucalyptus, juniper, orange, sandalwood, yarrow.

Liver- rosemary, peppermint, carrot seed, lemon, lavender, balm, mint.

Memory Aid - basil, clove, rosemary.

Muscle pain - rosemary, pine, marjoram, nutmeg, birch, meadowsweet.

Nervousness, stress - angelica, bergamot, balm, jasmine, clary, honey oil, neroli, sandalwood, coriander, ylang-ylang, cedar, tagetes, pine, basil, geranium, tarragon, galbanum, vetivert, rose, lavender.

Obesity - lemon, onion.

PMS - chamomile, galbanum, clary, neroli, ylang-ylang, marjoram.

Shock - camphor, coriander, mint, neroli.

Sinusitis - angelica, basil, pine, sandalwood, frankincense, marjoram, lavender, peppermint.

Skin diseases - rockrose, cedar, lemon, birch, geranium, carrot seed, pine, oregano, rose, onion (chapping), cajeput, chamomile, cade, sage.

Sore throat - bergamot, sandalwood, lemon, geranium, ginger, sage, thyme.

Sunburn - chamomile, lavender, yarrow.

Teething - chamomile.

Toothache - clove, cinnamon, cajeput, nutmeg, peppermint.

Urinary tract infections - cajeput, eucalyptus, fennel, geranium, juniper, lavender, lemon, niaouli, onion, pine, sage, thyme, savory.

Vomiting, nausea - mint, cajeput, dill, angelica, lemon, peppermint, aniseed, fennel.

Wounds - eucalyptus, cajeput, rockrose, chamomile, lavender, clove, rose, garlic, yarrow, hyssop, lemon, juniper, birch, rosemary, elemi, sage, geranium, savory, patchouly.

Ritual for Consecration of Oils in Healing and Magic

In the same way we consecrate all our magical tools to work for the betterment of life on earth, we also consecrate our magical oils.

Whether you purchase your scents or create your own, you should consecrate each single-note essence and every perfume blend you use, especially those that you set aside for anointing coveners, talismans, stones, or magical tools.

When you consecrate a single note fragrance you should focus on the quality of the flower or other parts of the botanical from which the scent has been extracted. The list of meanings of oils and incense ingredients in Appendix I explains these attributes. When you combine single notes into a perfume or aromatherapeutic blend, you must concentrate on the intent for which you have created this formula, for example; love for Aphrodite's Spell, prosperity for Midas, better health for Wings of Healing, success for Sun.

I like to store my oils in amber-colored one-ounce bottles topped with droppers. I also find it convenient to store everything in the same-size bottle, although the many beautiful and varied colors and shapes of bottles found on the market today are tempting.

I prefer my plain bottles not only for their conformity of size and shape but also because the dark color helps retard spoilage and the attached dropper makes the contents easy to use.

I have bought many new bottles in this shape and size, but have also recycled extract bottles from health food stores.

After pouring the oil and sealing the bottle, I wash the outside thoroughly in warm, soapy water, rinse well, and rub dry with a soft cloth. Then I label the bottle and place it on my altar until I find time to consecrate it.

During the consecration ritual I call upon Raschea, whom you met in chapter 2, and who is one of the 360 heads of the zone girdling the Earth. Allegedly these spirits hold all actions and conditions in a state of constant harmony. Raschea is associated with the fourth degree of Virgo. Franz Bardon in *The Practice of Magical Evocation* describes this angelic being:

> One could justly regard this head as the king of flowers,
> for all the flowers on our earth are under his protection.
> From this head the magician learns to understand the language

of flowers, i.e. the symbolic meanings of the various kinds of flowers in their relationship to man as well as to the universal laws. The colour, shape and number of the petals reveal to the magician the analogies to the universal laws and he sees from this what, in the world of flowers, is real beauty. Penetrating deeper into this knowledge the magician learns to look at and understand each flower from the esoteric point of view, and he learns to grasp the qualities of each flower in any respect and to use them for magic purposes. [12]

Preparation

When the moon is waxing and in Virgo, erect an altar, cover it with a white cloth, and prepare 2 white altar candles.

White is the combination of all the colors, and represents the myriad of scents in the world. Place an incense burner with coal and matches in the center of the altar next to the bottle of oil to be consecrated, and the candles on either side toward the back. You will light the coal during the rite, but you will not burn any incense. If there is a wall behind the altar, attach the sigil of Raschea (see chapter 2, figure 2.5) to the wall to contemplate during your meditation or to focus on when invoking. If there is no wall, draw the sigil on a stiff piece of cardboard and prop it up against a plate or book displayer. Bathe and don a white robe.

Meditation

Light the candles and sit before your altar meditating on Raschea's qualities and powers from the above description. Contemplate the seemingly ephemeral, but tenacious essence of scents, how they have always been on earth and will continue to permeate the atmosphere long after you have departed. Just imagine how the faint odor of incense was still distinguishable in King Tut's tomb when it was discovered many centuries after this Egyptian Pharaoh had been buried. Realize, too, how scent is one of the first things we perceive as we enter life, and how too, smell is the last sense that leaves us as we pass out of consciousness.

The Rite

When you are ready, stand facing East, and open the Circle by performing the Lesser Banishing and Invoking Pentagram Rituals or by using the Wicca Way. If you need help with these rituals, refer back to *Web of Light*.

Return to the altar and invoke Raschea:

"O Protector of the delicate flowers of this realm, that bring us good health, strength and joy, and without which our lives would be truly impoverished, I call upon you, Raschea, King of Flowers, to descend into this Circle of Light and instill this bottle of aromas with your mysterious potency. May I, under your guidance, penetrate the ancient secrets surrounding perfumes and use the knowledge thus obtained to improve the lives of humankind."

With your Athame trace a pentagram or a figure of a Celtic cross surrounded by a circle (figure 6.1) on the outside of the bottle. Say:

"By the power of the Mighty Ones and by Raschea, King of Flowers, I consecrate this bottle of aroma to help me work my magical aims to the glory of the Ineffable Name."

Now light the coal, uncap the bottle, and place a few drops of oil on the hot coal. Inhale deeply to incorporate some of the essence into your being. As you inhale and integrate the attributes of this oil, get to know the formula completely, and commit the scent to memory.

Recap the bottle, and close the Circle. Thank the Mighty Ones, and particularly the Spirit Raschea, for lending their power and protection to your ritual. The rite is ended. You can now add the oil to your healing arsenal.

Figure 6.1
Celtic Cross Surrounded by Circle

Appendix I
Perfume, Incense, and Potpourri Ingredients

ABSINTHE
(Artemisia absinthium)
Common Name: Wormwood
The leaves are used to flavor absinthe liqueur and vermouth. The plant is sacred to Isis, although in the Bible, it was driven out of the Garden of Eden. Add a pinch of the leaves to scrying incense, or incense for rituals to break up a love affair. This herb combines well in small amounts with sandalwood.

ACACIA
(Acacia senegal)
Common Name: Gum Arabic
The hard, close-grained wood of this tree, sacred to Osiris, is valued by cabinet makers. The wood is redolent of violets. Use the aromatic foliage and yellow flowers of this warm weather tree sparingly in love incenses or in petitions to the goddess. It is a favorite Buddhist fragrance. Anoint altar equipment with this solar-ruled oil. In the language of flowers acacia means "chaste love."

AGRIMONY
(Agrimonia eupatoria)
Common Name: Church Steeples

This Southern climate tree also goes by the name "country nun" because the flowers are shaped like the hand bells that some nuns used to carry in former times. The botanical is cultivated by the Chinese for its flowers that scent joss sticks. The yellow flower heads are a cedar substitute. During the Renaissance, the plant was considered a panacea. In the language of flowers, agrimony stands for "thankfulness."

ALLSPICE
(Pimenta officinalis, Eugenia pimenta)

Christopher Columbus discovered this tree and its spicy berries on one of his trips to the New World. He named it allspice because the aroma reminded him of a blend of cinnamon, clove, and nutmeg.

Add the spicy berries to incense and potpourri. Harvest the berries while they are green and fragrant, distill them in water for essential oil, and powder them for incenses. Use the berries whole or bruised in potpourris. The sweetly scented leaves also can be added to potpourris.

In occult perfumery, allspice draws success, develops will power and concentration, and improves school and work performance.

ALMOND
(Amygdalus communis)

Odorless sweet almond oil is a popular carrier for massage oils or for essential oils that must be ingested when the patient cannot tolerate a preparation diluted in alcohol. Bitter almond oil is extracted from the pellicle that covers the nut of the *A. amarga* after it has been shelled. The raw scent must be cut with alcohol in order to be pleasing. Its fruity scent, the hallmark of Jergen's Lotion, lends a velvety note to floral blends.

In the language of flowers the tree symbolizes "hope." The Arabs believed the oil contained the essence of love that conquers all adversity. The name in Hebrew means "early awakening."

In Greek legend, when Demophon was shipwrecked at Thrace, he fell in love with Phyllis, a king's daughter. When the warrior was called home on an emergency and did not return to his lover at their appointed date, she hanged herself. The gods changed the princess into a flowering almond tree. Because of Phyllis's youthful impetuosity, and sacrifice, in the language of flowers, almond signifies "indiscretion" and "the thoughtlessness of youth."

Add a few drops of the oil to Money-Draw incense when you need a lot of cash right away.

ALOE
(Lignum aloes)

The gum of this native African tree is a common incense ingredient. It is extracted from the leaves by incision. Aloe was used by Egyptians in embalming, Witches in Venusian incenses, and Black Magicians in incenses to increase their psychic powers and invoke demons. Alas, in the language of flowers this botanical stands for "grief" and "bitterness." The scent is associated with the High Priestess card in the tarot.

ALYSSUM
(Alyssum maritimum)
Common Name: Sweet Alyssum

The flowers make a wonderful potpourri ingredient with the delicate odor of new mown hay. The blooms last for a long time, and are not cut off until the first frost.

AMBER

The rich fragrance emitted by the pulverized fossil resin of extinct coniferous trees allegedly keeps a lover faithful and chases Witches and other negative influences from the home. Astrologers claim that it is worn well by extroverted, Leoine personalities. Witch healers employ it as a love oil and to balance and heal the aura because they believe the scent equalizes yin/yang extremes. An ancient love philtre calls for steeping amber in a bottle of red wine, and adding essence of rose, sandalwood, and ylang-ylang. On the Tree of Life, amber is associated with Hod, as well as with the god Mercury.

AMBERGRIS
(Sperm Whale)

This product of a disease in the intestinal tract of the sperm whale which forms from the whale's inability to digest cuttlefish, has been found in large globs floating on the sea. The biggest discovered piece measured 60 inches long and 30 inches in diameter. One pound of the wax can command more than $200 on the perfume market. The foul-smelling wax liquid turns deliciously honeyed and spicy when exposed to the air and when heavily distilled in alcohol.

French dandies in the eighteenth century carried pomanders scented with this essence, and Queen Elizabeth I scented her gloves with the voluptuous aroma. In the nineteenth century, boxes, stationery, and leather were permeated with ambergris because the fragrance is so long-lasting.

Ambergris is a fixative in perfumery, a love/sexual attraction oil, and sometimes is used as a flavoring in hot chocolate. Mix 4 parts ambergris, 2 parts musk, and 1 part vanilla for a dynamite attraction oil. According to Lady Sara, this scent is ruled by Pluto and Neptune.

ANGELICA
(Angelica officinalis, A. archangelica)
Common Name: Root of the Holy Ghost

The name of this six-foot tall botanical derives from its folk reputation as a remedy against plague, poison, enchantments, and mad dogs! The hardy botanical grows as far north as the Arctic Circle, so is available to many people around the world. In fact, at one time the Orientals revered the healing properties of the native Northern European plant in the same way that Occidentals prize ginseng today.

The essential oil of this umbelliferous celery-stalked herb is fragrantly musky and freshly peppery, and is used in perfumery, especially in Oriental and fern-like blends. Throw the seeds on the fire to fumigate the room. It is also a fixative in potpourri. As a carminative it is used in aromatherapy to strengthen the body. Burn the seeds in incense to repel evil.

ANISE
(Pimpinella anisum)
Common Name: Aniseed

One of the oldest fragrant seeds known to man, anise lends a spicy, licorice-like aroma to incenses such as Enchanted Forest, Vesta Fire, and formulas to improve clairvoyance and boost cerebral functions.

In aromatherapy anise is a remedy for flatulence, poor digestion, dizziness, heart palpitations, and painful menstruation. Imbibe as an infusion, 1 teaspoon per cupful of boiling water after meals. The oil also flavors gin, vermouth, and Chartreuse liqueur, and scents soap.

Laplanders believe that chewing the seeds increases the life span. Many Europeans bake anise into wedding cakes in the belief that it will bring good luck to the newlyweds.

APPLE BLOSSOM
(Malus genus)

This soft scent is thought to confer the wisdom of Aphrodite on the wearer and induce an ambience of peace and happiness in the home. In the language of flowers apple blossom means "preference," that is; it is "preferred" over rose because it is both a fruit and a flower. Apple blossom emits a light, airy, but long-lasting aroma.

APRICOT
(Prunus armeniaca)

Probably this was the actual apple of the Garden of Eden. The oil from inside the seed makes an effective emollient. The oil, nut, and fruit all supposedly increase the life span. Apricot lends a subtle, fruity fragrance to Satyr's Dance perfume.

BALM OF GILEAD

Many botanicals go by this name. The *Cedronella triphylla* is a shrub with fragrant leaves like a combination of lemon and coriander. *Abies balsamea*, also known as "balsam fir," is grown from Labrador to Iowa. It smells of spicy strawberries. In old times, housewives filled pillows with the lightly-scented leaves.

Commiphora opabalsamum, a small tree native to the Red Sea region, is the true balm of Gilead of old. Unfortunately, it is rare now.

The orangish-yellow, sticky buds of the *Populus balsamifera*, also called the poplar tree, have a delightfully heady aroma, and are an ingredient in healing incenses, as the botanical is associated with the sun. The Victorians recognized the curative value of balsam, and identified it with "relief from affliction" in the language of flowers. Added to the bath, this botanical helps beautify the skin.

Wear the buds in a sachet as an amulet for protection against hexes and to mend a broken heart. In the Bible, the Queen of Sheba brought Gilead buds to Judea as a present to King Solomon.

Steep the buds in wine, then dry them and wear them, or burn them in incense to draw love. Legend has it that if you coat your fingers with the sticky resin you can pass through fire without being burned.

BALSAM OF PERU
(Myroxylon balsamum var. *pereirae)*
The melliferous, vanilla-like oil comes from a resin obtained by burning a tall Central American (not Peruvian!) tree. It is used as a fixative in incenses and potpourris. M. toluiferum is another variety called balsam of Tolu. The perfume is an alleged hexbreaker, and is said to promote success in all endeavors and aid meditation.

BARBERRY
(Berberis vulgaris)
Add the bright red berries of this evergreen common to the Eastern United States to winter potpourris. The yellow flowers that hang in grape-like clusters in the springtime smell sour when fresh, but fragrant when dried. The language of flower meaning of this botanical aptly is "tartness."

BASIL
(Ocimum basilicum)

The common culinary spice (150 varieties exist, which is made from the crushed leaves of a bushy annual, gives a spicy, fresh aroma to Jupiter and Mars incenses. In the tarot, basil is linked to the Emperor trump. The name derives from a Greek word meaning "to smell strong." *O. sanctum* (holy basil) is sacred to Krishna and Vishnu in India, and is also known as the "herb of kings." Basil is associated with the fantastic beast, the basilisk, a reptile whose glance and breath are lethal.

Use both the dried leaves and seeds in cooking, potpourri, and Magic. In times gone by, basil was an ingredient of sweet waters, sweet bags, and nosegays.

Surround yourself with this aroma during meditation and ritual work when you wish to regenerate yourself and promote self-confidence, stability, leadership potential, achievement, and mental acuity. Legend claims that if you plant the seeds while muttering curses, the plant will thrive. The herb inexplicably means "hatred" in the language of flowers, even though it is associated with the sun, love, and prosperity.

In aromatherapy basil treats migraine headaches, gout, amenorrhea, and mental fatigue. Extract of basil is alleged to promote fertility. The pungent, peppery fragrance was claimed by Gerard "to remove melancholy and make men glad and happy."

Prepare an infusion of basil leaves by blending one tablespoon of the herb in a pint of water. Wash the doorknobs of your place of business and its threshold with the water to ward off vandals and thieves and attract business.

BAY
(Laurus nobilis)
California Laurel
(Umbellularia californica)

The bay laurel is sacred to Apollo. The perfume extracted from the leaves and berries of this evergreen native to Southern Europe is tangy, and blends well with spicy, citrusy scents, and carnation. The dominant note in Bay Rum toiletries comes from the *Pimenta acris*, the "bay rum" or "black cinnamon" tree, as it is known in the West Indies. In aromatherapy, bay leaves join forces with eucalyptus in the battle to help cure the common cold.

This balsamic, spicy scent allegedly draws love, psychic visions, and insures victory for athletes. It fulfills wishes, and protects the home. The finely ground leaves in sandalwood incense repel the negative influences of Saturn. Bay stands for "glory" in the language of flowers.

In Witchcraft, the fresh fragrance keeps poltergeists, Witches and fleas (!) "at bay." A leaf burned in an incense or added to a meat dish is said to draw power and wealth. In *The Faerie Queen* Edmund Spenser calls bay "the mead of mighty conquerors."

BENZOIN
(Stryax benzoin)
Common Names: Gum Benjamin, Benjamin Tree

The sweet-smelling, grayish-brown or reddish resin is obtained from the fuzzy bark of a tree native to the East Indies, China, Java, and Sumatra. A vanilla-scented variety hailing from Sri Lanka is quite popular burned as incense. The resin also makes a fragrant fixative for oils, potpourris, and sachets. The odor harmonizes with geranium, orange blossom, and rose.

According to C.W. Septimus Piesse in the classic nineteenth century work, The Art of Perfumery, benzoin "forms a good basis for a bouquet. Like balsam of Tolu, it gives permanence and body to a perfume made with an essential oil in spirit." [13]

In aromatherapy, benzoin is a stimulant and antiseptic when taken externally in a tincture, and a carminative, diuretic, and mild expectorant when ingested. Tincture of benzoin, which is inexpensive and readily available in drugstores, can be mixed with steaming water as an inhalant for laryngitis, croup, and bronchitis. In a lotion it soothes chapped skin. The botanical reputedly ameliorates discharges of various kinds. Inhale benzoin tincture and lavender essence to revive yourself from psychic and physical exhaustion.

Magically, benzoin reputedly drives away evil spirits, promotes self-growth, grants prayers, induces visions, and persuades spirits. Burn the powdered resin in purification rites. A combination of benzoin, sandalwood, and rose makes a love oil supreme.

BERGAMOT
(Citrus bergamia)

Expressed from the peel of the bitter, yellow, pear-shaped fruit of a citrus tree native to Italy, this green essential oil lends its strikingly rich aroma to Earl Grey tea. Add it to hip baths to relieve muscular tension. It is a vaginal douche, effective against bladder infections and ingested as a nerve tonic that also alleviates pain from cancer of the uterus, tumors, and intestinal cramps. The essential oil is an antiseptic for eczema, an antispasmodic, and vermifuge. In aromatherapy, bergamot heightens levels of concentration, stimulates the mind, and prevents fatigue.

It combines well as a top note with lavender, orange blossom and other citrus scents, jasmine, and cypress. Bergamot is one of the ingredients of *Eau de Cologne*, which was the first mixed bouquet perfumiers ever concocted. It was created in Cologne, Germany in the eighteenth century by the famous Italian perfumier, Feminis. In occult perfumery, bergamot repels evil and psychic attack when rubbed in the palm of the hand, or when used to anoint candles. The oil also protects a person from physical damage, so it is a choice anointing oil for travel protection talismans.

Monarda fistulosa and *M. didyma*, an herb plant also called bergamot, bee balm, or Oswego tea, is used in perfumery, especially in sweet waters. When added to the bath, it is supposed to help alleviate joints painfully swollen from arthritis. The leaves are very sweetly scented with a touch of pepperiness. American Indians and feisty American colonists during the Boston Tea Party era commonly drank Oswego tea in protest against the English tea tax. (Also see ORANGE BLOSSOM, PETTIGRAIN.)

BIRCH BARK
(Betula alba, B. lenta, B. negra.)
Common Name: Lady of the Wood

The chips of this bark make a reasonable substitute for pine in incense. The leaves and bark of the black birch (*B. lenta*) render an aromatherapeutic oil redolent of wintergreen. In fact, since true oil of wintergreen is no longer manufactured, products labelled with wintergreen as an ingredient are either birch oil or salicylate. In aromatherapy, birch is an ingredient in liniments and unguents that relieves arthritis and sore muscles and cleans wounds. It is also a lymphatic drawer.

In the language of flowers birch stands for "gracefulness" and "meekness." It is said that the tree acquired this meaning because it is an undemanding, yet slenderly beautiful tree. It is also very hardy and a symbol of the return of spring in Northern climes. Carry a piece of birch bark in a mojo bag to protect yourself from enchantments.

BISTORT
(Polygonum bistorta)
Common Names: Dragonwort, Snakeweed

Eat the young leaves like spinach. Bistort root is touted to alleviate heavy menstrual bleeding. Add it to incense to promote psychic visions.

BLOODROOT
(Sanguinaria canadensis)
Common Names: Indian Paint, Red Puccoon, Redroot,
Tetterwort

This poisonous botanical found in woods, fields, and on river banks tastes nauseating. The fleshy root was used by American Indians as a dye. It is identified by its single white flower and pale green, lobed leaf which sprouts from the reddish-orange rhizome.

The roots are a cathartic, expectorant, emmenagogue, and emetic. In folk medicine the plant was used to cure bronchitis, dyspepsia, asthma, ringworm, eczema, skin cancer, and fungal growths. I do not recommend you prescribe it medicinally because it is strongly emetic and lowers the pulse rate dangerously. The root is so caustic it corrodes tissue.

Appropriately, bloodroot is associated with Mars, the warrior god of the North American Indians. It's main magical virtue is in incense-burning as an amulet against evil spirits. Throw the burning herb on an enemy's doorstep to turn back wicked spells. Burn the powdered root for seven nights at midnight to purify your dwelling. Sprinkle it in an unbroken circle around your house to keep evil from gaining entry.

BROOM

(Genista tinctoria, Cytisus scoparius)

Common Names: Scotch Broom, Irish Broom

Contrary to the geographical implications of this botanical's common names, most of the essence used in perfumery comes from France (*C. purgans*). *Genista* is a fragrant native of Sicily, much favored by bees.

The tips of the broom plant are poisonous, but nonetheless the yellow flowers are used in Mars incense. Perhaps because of its toxicity it was cursed in the Bible. The legend goes that the leaves crackled when Mary and Joseph fled into Egypt, thereby revealing their whereabouts to Herod's soldiers.

The flower stands for "humility" and "neatness" in the language of flowers, probably because the stems were gathered and often fashioned into crude brooms by peasants. This flower also claims a more elevated association, as it was taken as the badge of King Henry II of England. In fact, the entire royal line of Plantagenet derives from one of the Latin names for this botanical. The perfume is alleged to bring joy and luck to the home, and helps focus the mind in meditation.

CAJEPUT

(Melaleuca leucadendron)

Common Names: White Tea Tree, Swamp Tea Tree

This native of the Australian, Malaysian, Indian and Phillipine forests is believed to ward off illness. Bathe in the essence expressed from the leaves and buds to cure scratches, sore muscles, headache, and frostbite. Cajeput releases a camphor-like aroma that is effective in therapeutic massage oil. Internally, the essence is a general antiseptic, calmative, and vermifuge. In aromatherapy, this analgesic and bronchial decongestant cures ear and toothaches.

CALAMUS

(Acorus calamus)

Common Names: Sweet Flag, Sweet Sedge, Sweet Grass

This lusciously fruity addition for potpourris is mentioned frequently in the Old Testament as an incense ingredient, where often it is confused with citronella grass. The powdered root, when added to Graveyard Dust, produces a controlling incense. Calamus contains fixative properties. The cut root lends a pleasant aroma to incense. The fragrance is prized in perfumery for its vanilla-like aroma. The Indian variety is highly toxic; do not ingest.

CAMPHOR GUM
(Cinnamomum camphora)

Easily recognized for its odor of mothballs, camphor has a clean and pungent smell similar to eucalyptus. Camphor is distilled from the leaves and wood chips of a tree native to South China, Formosa, and Japan, and naturalized in California. The durable wood once was carved into storage chests for sailors to keep their clothing insect-free.

The gum is employed in lunar incense recipes, and is associated with the High Priestess card in the tarot. Lady Sara says the gum is a psychic energizer. I recommend care in using camphor in aromatherapy, as it is a dangerous excitant in large doses.

CARAWAY
(Carum carvi)

The name in Old English means "care-away," and refers to the seed's soothing redolence when burned. The botanical is linked with Mercury and Saturn.

Caraway is a common culinary herb of the carrot family, similar to anise, dill, and fennel. The plant grows two-feet tall with white or yellow flowers and feathery, dusty green or turquoise leaves. The herb's long, tapered root, often confused with deadly water hemlock, is an aromatic in incenses. Since Roman times, caraway has flavored cookies, bread, cake, soup, cabbage, cheese, and Kummel liqueur.

It is a carminative and mild stimulant to the digestion. Powder the seeds and make a poultice to reduce swelling from bruises. Chewing caraway seeds helps relieve intestinal gas. It is also used as a dentifrice.

Be sure the seeds are absolutely dry before harvesting, or they will turn fetid. Burn caraway at home in protection incense to prevent your possessions from being stolen. Allegedly the seeds keep mates faithful and reveal if a lover is telling the truth; so caraway makes a useful component of some love incenses. It can also be ground into a sachet. The scent combines well with lavender and clove.

If you own poultry, feed them caraway seeds to keep them from straying from the barnyard. Sew seeds into a small bag, and stuff it in your baby's pillow for protection.

CARDAMOM
(Elettaria cardamomum)
The hot, spicy, reddish-brown seeds are known throughout the Arab world as an aphrodisiac. They blend well with almost any incense. The seeds also season breads and coffee.

CARNATION
(Dianthus genus)
Common Name: Gillyflower
The name is a corruption of "coronation," because in the old days carnations were worn in chaplets and coronets. Another of its names, dianthus, means "flower of the gods."

Some of the snappiest scented blooms hail from Colorado, although for perfume, the best quality blossoms are said to come from Southern France. In general, the red varieties are more heavily perfumed than the white or yellow. This fragrance mixes well with clove, clary sage, lavender, lily-of-the-valley, narcissus, rose, and ylang-ylang.

Aromatherapists claim that this stimulant restores energy and promotes healing. In Merrie Olde England, tincture of carnation was an ingredient of medicinal syrups.

Carnations symbolize femininity, gentle love, allurement, and fidelity. The flower was chosen by Miss Jarvis, the inventor of Mothers' Day, to honor all mothers. From that time forward, carnations have represented motherly love. In the language of flowers, this botanical means "fascination" and "women's love." It is the birth flower of January.

According to myth, people of religious inclination are attracted to white carnations, and those who crave to do things in a grandiose manner are drawn to the red variety. Witches use the oil to anoint and consecrate their incense burners and many ritual tools. They also inhale it to restore their energies after performing healing rites.

In Korean legend if you adorn your hair with three carnations on a single stem, and the bottom flower dies first, you will have troubles early in life. If the top flower dies first, your later years will be difficult. If all three die at once, you will be unlucky all your life! Moral of the story: if you don't adorn your hair with carnations, maybe you will avoid bad luck!

CASCARILLA
(Eluteria genus)
Common Name: Sweet Bark

Add the bark of this small tree native to the Bahamas to incenses to achieve a musky fragrance. Cascarilla assimilates well in earthy incenses. The highly fragrant, white flowers unfortunately are not used in perfumery. The botanical is thought to be a source of power.

CASSIA
(Cinnamomum cassia, Cassia fistula)

The bark of this tree smells like cinnamon, and was burned by ancient Greeks, Romans, Arabs, Chinese, and Indians in their temples and homes to protect them, promote psychic dreams, draw positive influences, and bring happiness. Cassia is also alleged to increase sexual desire.

In fragrance blending cassia ranks as an inferior substitute for cinnamon. It often finds its way into potpourris because of its low price.

CASTOREUM

This substance collected from the glands of beavers is distilled in spirits of wine to produce its distinctive odor. It is easily recognizable as the signature scent of Russian leather. The oil is used in rites of Saturn.

CAYENNE
(Capiscum annum)

Add this familiar red, hot, culinary pepper sparingly to incenses and sachets to make things happen or to drive away unwanted guests, neighbors, and bosses. It is a key ingredient of Voodoo Hotfoot Powder.

CEDAR
(Cedrus libani; C. atlantica; Juniperus virginiana - red cedar)
Common Name: Oil of the Unicorn

The name derives from an Arabic word meaning "something of great value." *C. atlantica*, now grown only in Morocco, was probably the Tree of Life in the Bible, described as containing the secret power of longevity. The wood was used to build the Temple of Solomon. According to one source, only a few hundred trees are still extant. *J. virginiana* and *J. mexicana*, types of juniper similar in scent to cedar, are used extensively in the American perfume industry because they are so much less expensive than Moroccan cedar.

Cedar was an Egyptian mummification ingredient also used to impregnate papyrus leaves in order to keep hieroglyphic manuscripts safe from the ravages of insects in the same way it protects clothes in our closets today. The wood went into building Egyptian temples, ships coffins, furniture, and palaces. In aromatherapy, it can be inhaled to alleviate bronchial congestion, and is applied externally as an antiseptic and to stimulate hair growth. Do not ingest the essential oil during pregnancy.

In small amounts, cedar elicits a fresh, woody aroma from rose, juniper, sandalwood, vetivert, violet, patchouly, and cypress. To make tincture of cedar, steep the chips in spirits and filter. The sawdust in potpourri and incense lends a tangy, resinous fragrance. Like all conifers, the odor of cedar is said to soothe the nervous and respiratory systems.

Cedar is associated with majesty, royalty, and grandeur, and is ruled by Jupiter. In Magic, the oil consecrates wands, invokes Odin, instills the Magician with confidence, and insures a long, well-protected life.

CHAMOMILE
(Anthemis nobilis - Roman chamomile)
(Chamomilla Matricaria - German Chamomile)

The daisy-like flower of this delicate-looking herb is one of the oldest English herbal remedies. Its tonic fragrance combines well with rose, geranium, and lavender, and makes a superior ingredient in solar, healing, and Winter Solstice incenses. It is also a blessing oil in rituals to draw money.

Because it grew in the pathways of pilgrims, who when stepping on it released its fragrance in the air, it was quipped that "the camomile shall teach the patience that rises best when trodden upon." Perhaps this is why in the language of flowers, chamomile stands for "energy in adversity" and "humility."

The foliage of German chamomile serves as a festive background in bouquets while the showy white flowers of Roman chamomile are perfect for potpourri. *Matricaria matricariodes,* otherwise known as manzanilla or pineapple weed, gives off an apple-scented aroma, and the leaves often are confused with true chamomile.

In aromatherapy chamomile provides a valuable remedy as an analgesic, aperitif, analgesic, cholagogue, hypnotic, stimulant, and stomachic. It assuages the pain from colitis and gastritis when taken internally, and in a poultice for shingles, eczema, and abscesses. Chamomile tea eases the cramps associated with difficult menstruation. Strain an infusion of the flowers, and apply to blond hair to add highlights and keep it shiny. The essence is alleged to help a person overcome melancholy and anger.

CHERRY
(Prunus serotina)

This cheerful essence is distilled from the sweet pink and white blossoms of the cherry tree. The fragrance is alleged to encourage light-hearted activities, and a gay, carefree environment. In the language of flowers, the blossom means "education." The wood of the choke cherry (*P. virginiana*) is a popular Needfire ingredient. Do not gather and store too much cherry wood at a time as it spoils rapidly.

CINNAMON
(Cinnamomum zeylanicum)

The oil, taken from the inner bark of a native Indian tree, composes part of the Egyptian embalming and anointing oils, and at one time was considered more valuable than gold.

It is alleged to awaken sexuality, and is a primary ingredient in love potions. Yet the energy it imparts is of a peaceful nature, so it is an excellent oil with which to bless a room. Only add a few drops when blending cinnamon oil into a perfume because it can irritate the skin and the spiciness overpowers more delicate fragrances. It harmonizes with jasmine, lime, tonka, and ylang-ylang. Cinnamon aids creativity and concentration when combined with sandalwood.

Add the granules to potpourri to lend a piquant note. In ancient times, cinnamon was burned in temples to offset the stench of burnt offerings. In the same vein, a cinnamon-like potpourri or sachet in the kitchen will do wonders to disperse the smell of culinary sacrifices.

The powder ground from the bark is reputed to invoke the gods, bring fast luck, and aid the memory when added to incense. Burn cinnamon incense at the dinner table in order to help maintain a happy home. Cinnamon is also an ingredient of solar incenses.

In aromatherapy and herbal medicine, cinnamon is valued as an antiseptic, astringent, antispasmodic, aphrodisiac, parasiticide, and heart tonic. Eighty drops of essence added to one quart of water is said to help the above conditions. A delicious aphrodisiac wine is concocted with cinnamon by combining 600 drops each of vanilla, ginseng, rhubarb and cinnamon, and adding the mixture to 1 quart of chilled white wine.

CINQUEFOIL
(Potentilla reptans, P. anserina)
Common Name: Five Fingers Grass

This creeping perennial is burned in protection and offertory incenses to gain favors. It is a favorite Voodoo herb for banishing negativity and imbalance.

CITRONELLA
(Cymbopogon schoenanthus, C. nardus)
Common Name: Citronella Grass

A pungent, citrusy essential oil from Central America, Malaysia, China, and Sri Lanka, citronella is a valuable rinse for oily hair and skin and drives away insects from the picnic table. *C. Schoenanthus* renders Indian geranium oil. In Magic, anoint letters and all writing materials with it because it is thought to confer eloquence. The scent also restores peace and harmony to the home -- maybe because it drives away all those bugs!

CIVET
(Viverra civetta)
Civet is extracted from the gland under the tail of a wildcat raised in captivity in Sri Lanka, India, and Africa. The concentrated essence is most foul smelling—something like a combination of sweaty feet, mouldy cheese, and a dead rat -- but once the oil is diluted many times, it exudes a delicate, musky odor. The cats are raised specifically so they can be milked of the essence, and although they are not killed, the extraction process is painful for

them. For this reason, I recommend you buy only synthetic civet oil.

Civet is a fixative in perfumery. As an anointing oil for the breasts, it acts to attract love. Apply it to your feet for spiritual guidance.

CLARY SAGE
(Salvia sclarea)

Clary sage is a tall, graceful plant similar to ordinary sage with velvety oval leaves and pale blue or lilac flowers. "Clary" derives from the Latin term, *clarus,* meaning "clear," which refers to its alleged healing benefits for strengthening the eyes, stomach, uterus, kidneys, and back. It is good to use throughout a pregnancy and to help anyone who is engaged in creative pursuits, but epileptics should stay away from the oil because it exercises a strong effect on the central nervous system.

The oil is a nerve tonic that imparts a feeling of euphoria and peacefulness. It is also an ingredient of Muscatel wine. The lavender-scented perfume is used as a fixative in potpourri. Clary mixes harmoniously with bergamot, cypress, geranium, jasmine, lavender, orange, and sandalwood oils. In the Occult clary sage is a well regarded protection and visionary oil. In Gem Magic it is associated with the opal.

CLOVE
(Caryophyllus aromaticus, Eugenia caryophyllata)

The unopened buds of this aromatic evergreen native to the Moluccas was used liberally in the nineteenth century as a purifying essence for handkerchiefs, and earlier in sponges for plague victims. Later it was discovered that clove essence kills typhoid germs.

Clove is a respected aphrodisiac that also acts as a fixative when combined with orris. The strong fragrance tends to overpower more tenacious scents, but even so, combines well with carnation, citrus, cinnamon, and geranium. It is enjoyed as a breath freshener, mouthwash, and toothache alleviator.

Use clove oil aromatherapeutically for headaches, deafness, and to prepare the body for childbirth. A single clove preserves beef for 24 hours. English smelling salts rely on a mixture of cloves, cinnamon, lavender, camphor, and aniseed.

Whole, bruised, and powdered buds add a warm, cleanly spicy aroma to solar incense and potpourris.

The scent allegedly induces astral visions. As mentioned above, the clove tree is a native of the Moluccas where it was so admired that the nobility were rated according to whether they were worth one, two, three or four cloves. Thus the scent has come to signify "dignity" in the language of flowers.

CLOVER
(*Trifolium pratense* - Red Clover)
(*T. repens* - White Clover)

The name derives from an old Anglo-Saxon word meaning "club of Hercules." The tripartite leaf is also the model for the playing cards' suit of Clubs.

In Magic, clover represents good fortune and faithfulness. Place a few drops on your loved one's pillow each night to insure fidelity. Clover allegedly dissolves mischievous fairy spells. To dream of a field of clover presages wealth and prosperity. Carry a few flowers when you travel to insure a safe journey.

In the language of flowers, this honey-like blossom means "industry," an apt name, as all summer long, clover is assaulted by "busy bees."

During the pre-Revolutionary era, housewives dried the blossoms and lay them in the linen closets as a sweetener. Red clover makes a pretty addition to potpourris.

The following Old English rhyme shows another use for clover:

> A clover, a clover or two,
> Put in your right shoe,
> The first young man you meet
> In field, street or lane,
> You'll have him or one of his name.

COCONUT
(*Palmaceae*)

The scent pressed from the oil of this fruit of a palm tree signifies strength in adversity. It is used in Aquarian blends.

COPAL
(Copalli)
Common Name: Copalqua huitl

This prized Mexican black or white resin is obtained from different trees of the same genus. The white varieties are more expensive. Copal is also gathered in India, Madagascar, Mozambique and Zanzibar. The sensual fragrance calls upon the Horned God in his Pan or Cernunnos aspects. Copal also blends well in Native American incenses.

CORIANDER
(Coriandrum sativum)
Common Name: Cilantro

The foul-smelling fruit (often called a seed) of this umbelliferous herb releases a pleasant, flowery scent when dried. It is used in herbal medicine and in aromatherapy (take 3 drops of the essence in honey water after meals), as a carminative, and stomachic. It is claimed that the juice from the fresh plant affects the human organism like alcohol in that it initially excites, then depresses. It is supposed to eliminate stress and irritability.

The ancient book of tales, *The Arabian Nights*, recommends burning whole or crushed coriander seeds in love incenses. Try blending a few drops of the extract into love perfumes.

The herb means "concealed merit" in the language of flowers. It was a prime ingredient of the Carmelite nuns' famed *Eau de Paris* of the seventeenth century.

CORNFLOWER
(Centaurea cyanus)
Common Names: Bachelor's Button, Blue Bottle

This soft-hued, blue flower is called "delicacy" in the language of flowers. In Greek mythology, Cyanus loved the flower so much he wandered through cornflower fields, fashioning wreaths from the blue flowers, and clothing himself in them. When the goddess Flora found him dead in a field, she felt such compassion she transformed him into a cornflower.

Cornflower oil is alleged to aid clairvoyance and enhance creative powers. The bright blue flowers are lovely in potpourri.

CUBEB

(Piper cubeba)

The spicy berries are intensely aromatic and have been employed by the Arabs for centuries in love spells. They also can be inhaled by asthmatics either in incense or in cigarettes. In *Magical Charms, Potions and Secrets for Love*, C.A. Nagle recommends that men drink the ground powder mixed in a sweet beverage or with honey to arouse the passions and facilitate an erection [14].

CYPRESS

(Cupressus sempervirens)

This majestic, conical-shaped tree found principally in graveyards in this country, but originating in the Himalayas, symbolizes "the immortal soul." It is associated with Saturn, the planet of practicality, and Naña, the grandmother goddess of the Brazilian pantheon. Cypress reminds us to organize our thoughts in order to make our dreams realities. The woodsy-spicy, balsamic scent is definitely yang, and often is liked by Aquarian natives or anyone who seeks the universal.

The essence obtained from the leaves and fruit calms excitable children when rubbed on the throat and forehead. The oil constricts blood vessels when applied externally, so is good for varicose veins, and treats bleeding of the uterus and groin, all kinds of hemorrhages, bronchitis, and emphysema. Inhale cypress vapors to cure stuffy sinuses. Some have touted it as an anticancer medication. The essential oil is antiseptic and astringent, and can be used as a body deodorizer and antiperspirant. To alleviate hemorrhoids, combine 20 drops of cypress essence with 100 drops of balm of poplar (one of the balms of Gilead). Add a few drops to dandruff and oily hair shampoos.

In perfumery, cypress blends well with cedar, citrus, labdanum, lavender, pine, and sandalwood.

A symbol of mourning for the dead, cypress also blesses the living with its calm, masculine, spiritual essence. In Gem Magic it is associated with onyx.

DAPHNE
(Daphne mezereum, D. alpina, D. caucasica)

A hardy, deciduous shrub with fragrant, white, pink, or purple flowers redolent of lilacs, daphne is a native of the European Alps. The flowers are highly valued in perfumery for their sunny fragrance. *D. laureola* is most strongly scented at dusk.

DATURA
(Datura stramonium)

In perfumery this is not the rank-smelling jimson weed (*D. stramonium*) that rears its spiny heads in garbage dumps and wastelands, but *D. cornucopia, D. ceraticaula,* and *D. meteloides,* which emit heavenly fragrances. Datura flowers display long, white trumpets.

Unfortunately, all parts of the datura plant are extremely poisonous. It is said that two seeds inhaled in incense produce psychedelic trips, four seeds, madness, and that six seeds will kill. Even a whiff of the *D. stramonium* can produce headaches and dizziness. It is an ingredient of the ancient Witches Flying Ointment. While I do not recommend its use in incense, the fragrant essential oils from the sweet-smelling datura flowers seem harmless in perfumery unless they are ingested.

DEERS' TONGUE
(Trilisa odoratissima)

The leaves of this plant smell like vanilla and are used to improve the aroma of tobacco and potpourri. In Voodoo the leaves are added to incense to call upon the great god, Damballah. Witches include the leaves in incenses to bring peace to the home.

DITTANY OF CRETE
(Origanum dictananus)

An important ingredient in Earth incenses, it encourages manifestations. Dion Fortune devised a formula using equal parts of dittany, benzoin, sandalwood, and vanillan powders for astral travel. In the language of flowers this plant represents "birth," and is sacred to the goddess, Lucina, mother of Juno, who "brings forth into the light."

The Mercury ruled botanical is related to marjoram, and can be interchanged with marjoram (*O. marjoranum*) or oregano (*O.*

vulgare) in incense formulas. This is important because it is difficult anymore to find a supplier of dittany. On the Tree of Life, dittany is associated with Malkuth.

DRAGON'S BLOOD
(Daemonorops draco, Calamus draca)

This resin exudes from the fruit of a tropical tree found in Sumatra and Borneo. It is said to bring back loved ones when burned. Use it in Mars incenses to add a pungent, but sweet note, or to color magical ink. It is also a cosmetics ingredient. Combine dragon's blood with aloes and cinnamon powder, and add to Inner Temple incense to encourage prophetic dreams.

ELEMI
(Canarium luzonicum)

A balsamic, camphor-like gum from Brazil and the Phillipines that is used as a fixative in perfumery and as an ingredient for medicinal unguents and balms.

EUCALYPTUS
(Eucalyptus citriodora, E. globulus)
Common Name: Silver Dollar Tree

The crushed leaves of this Australian native tree are a popular incense and potpourri ingredient because they lend a camphor-like but also brightly citrusy aroma. The *citriodora* variety smells lemony, and the *stuartiana* variety smells like apples. For some strange reason, many potpourri ingredient suppliers dye the soft, green-colored leaves a bright green or pink color unknown in nature. If you use small amounts of eucalyptus in potpourri I suggest you buy the undyed leaves from a culinary spice supplier; you will appreciate the naturally beautiful results.

Eucalyptus is a powerful germicide. Inhale the essence, or combine it with 10 drops of pure thyme and lavender oil in a steaming bowl of water to clear your sinuses and reduce coughing from asthma, pulmonary tuberculosis, and the flu. The decidedly yang fragrance combines well with lavender, lemon verbena, and pine.

Eucalyptus is used magically as an anointing and purification oil.

FENNEL
(Foeniculum vulgare)

The seeds from this botanical, which taste and smell like anise, flavor many fish dishes. When burned, fennel reputedly lengthens the lifespan and shields a person from vice. During Medieval times, homeowners hung the whole herb from their doorways to repel evil.

It is an appropriate herb in Virgoan incenses, as it relieves the indigestion and flatulence to which many people born under that star sign are prone, and helps suppress the appetite for dieters. Roman gladiators mixed fennel in their food as a stimulant; so in the language of flowers, it came to represent "strength" and "heroism." Fennel is the signature ingredient of Psychic Vision and other clairvoyant incenses.

FEVERFEW
(Chrysanthemum parthenium, Tomacetum parthenium)
Common Name: Featherfew

The close-growing, white heads that look like Roman chamomile, add color and bulk, but not scent to potpourri. Plant a stand near the house to purify the air and keep flies away.

FIR
(Abies balsamea)

This stately tree grows to a height of 100 feet with one 450-foot specimen living in the Sierra Nevada. Significantly, in the language of flowers, fir means "elevation." Fir claims first place as North America's favorite Christmas tree. Add the needles to incenses to invoke the power of the god, or when you wish to create a visionary formula. The essence distilled from the branches alleviates genito-urinary tract infections.

FRANGIPANI
(Plumeria alba. P. rubra)

The oil, in former times known as "the eternal perfume," expressed from the delicately fragrant leaves of this native West Indian botanical allegedly draws love, psychic vibrations, harmony, admiration, and trust. Traditionally, it is worn by confidants.

The aroma of frangipani is redolent of gardenia and honeysuckle. When the sailors aboard Columbus's ships caught a whiff of its heady fragrance, they knew that land was near.

FRANKINCENSE
(Boswellia carterii)
Common Name: Olibanum

This universally popular incense ingredient substitutes for any other gum in incense-making. In ancient times, frankincense was as important to international commerce and politics as oil is today. Its spicy, woodsy, light fragrance blends well with rose and oriental-type scents. Frankincense provides a strong base note for almost any blend.

The scent allegedly drives away evil spirits and impure thoughts, and draws the spiritual serenity of the Light. It also attracts money and success, answers prayers, and binds spells. The cleansing attributes of frankincense naturally fumigate the sick room. Burning the resin supposedly frees one from such vile (!) habits as overeating. In aromatherapy, frankincense is valued for its ability to shrink breast inflammations and treat uterine troubles, sinusitis, and colds. It is an antiseptic and astringent as well.

Henri Gamache in *The Magic of Herbs* relates the following legend about the origin of frankincense:

> Leucothea who was a daughter of a Persian king was wooed and won by the God, Apollo. The king in order to avenge his stained honor ordered his daughter burned alive. Although Apollo was unable to save his lover's life, he sprinkled nectar and ambrosia over her grave which seeped through her body changing it into a beautiful tree which exudes a sap which becomes transformed into resinous tears. These are sold commercially as Olibanum Tears. [15]

GALANGAL
(Alpinia officinarum)
Common Name: Chewing John

Galangal is a spicy ingredient of Egyptian Kyphi incense. It also is burned in High John the Conqueror incenses, and is carried for good luck and invincibility.

GALBANUM
(Ferrula galbanifera)
This gum with the odor of fresh green peppers that only used to be available from Arabia, is a superior fixative in perfumery that lends a sassy, green note to blends. In aromatherapy it is known as a curative for female complaints.

Galbanum incense calms troubled waters, enhances spirituality, and purifies the Circle. In folklore galbanum was touted to drive away serpents and protect the home. It is also employed in the varnish-making process.

GARDENIA
(Gardenia florida, G. jasminoides)
Also known as cape jasmine, the perfume extracted from the gardenia's white flowers vibrates love pure and sweet. Unfortunately, as with most white flowers, the beautiful blossoms do not dry well for potpourris.

Occultly, it is a protective oil that nixes hexes, and is a key ingredient of Spirit perfume. Anoint a white candle with it to keep your lover from leaving you.

GERANIUM
(Pelargonium genus; P. robertianum - Herb-robert*)*
Common Name: Herb-robert
The cheerful window box flower from which a refreshing essence is distilled is a native of Algeria, Guinea, Thailand, and Reunion. The most fragrant blooms are alleged to come from Madagascar. The scent combines well with bergamot, clove, heliotrope, lemon verbena, lavender, musk, patchouly, vanilla, and rose. At one time, over two hundred varieties existed in Great Britain. Eventually, the scentless zonal geranium with its huge blossoms caught the public's fancy and was cultivated to the exclusion of other varieties. This has been a sad loss to the world of perfumery.

American Indians relied on a wild geranium (*Geranium maculatum* - Cranesbill) as a method of birth control. It supposedly reduces yin/yang extremes, calms the nerves, aids the transition through menopause, and is a good antiseptic and mosquito repellant. In the early 1960's several species of geranium were found to possess anticoagulant properties.

The fragrance is worn by those of a daring, active, unconventional, sexual nature. It is an ingredient in magical floor washes to protect and purify the home. Anoint altars and personal possessions with geranium oil, and use it to break hexes. Wear it when those who are jealous of your success begin to spread gossip about you -- their viciousness will backfire on them.

A few dried leaves or flowers lend an exotic aroma to any incense or potpourri. Some varieties have unusual scents like lemon, nutmeg, musk, orange, rose, lavender, apple, spice, cinnamon, filbert, lemon, and violet. The rose-scented variety (*P. capitatum, P. radula*) so closely approximates the fragrance of real roses that it was used by the unscrupulous for years to adulterate the more expensive attar of rose.

In the language of flowers, scented geraniums hold different meanings: lemon for an unexpected meeting, nutmeg for an expected meeting, oak-leaved for true friendship, rose for preference, and scarlet for comfort.

GINGER
(Zingiber officinale)
Common Name: Roscoe

A spicy fragrance known to Western medicine and cookery since the Middle Ages but used in the Orient for much longer, ginger root brightens the day. I find that candied ginger and Lipton's ginger tea aid my digestion. Apply the perfume oil to your temples when leaving home to open the door to an exciting, romantic time.

Wild ginger (*Asarum canadense*) is distilled from the leaves of a creeping dwarf plant, and combines well with Pikaki to make Rising Moon oil. Offer whole ginger root to the elemental spirits.

GORSE
(Ulex europeus)
Common Names: Furze, Whin

As an Old English saying goes, "When gorse is out of blossom kissing's out of fashion." This hardy, shrubby, spiny little bush with cheery yellow flowers that always smell sweetly of springtime and honey brightens the British countryside all year 'round.

Monks, who since the sixth century have lived on the Isle of Caldey off Tenby in Southwest Wales, make the most delightfully melliferous gorse perfume. If you are in Britain, it is well worth a trip to the island to buy some. In the language of flowers, the plant aptly stands for "endless affection."

GRAINS OF PARADISE
(Aframomum melgueta)
These seeds bring luck, money, love and protection when added to incense, or when enclosed with other items in a mojo bag. According to Voodoo, this botanical is an all-around improver of conditions. Add the grains to love potion wine to stimulate desire.

GRAPE
(Vitis genus)
Believers in Voodoo swear the fragrance pulls in money and popularity, and removes curses. The scent is all-pervasive and long-lasting.

HEATHER
(Calluna vulgaris)
The light, airy fragrance is distilled from a low-growing plant of the Heath family, native to Scotland, where it blooms in countless varieties. Its genus name in Greek means "to sweep," as the branches once were used as brooms. *Phyllodoce breweri*, another kind of heather, is an antibacterial, and is used to subtly color dried flower arrangements.

Heather is alleged to bring long life and immortality, keep loneliness at bay, and increase one's personal beauty. It is worn by those on the path of Wicca to "light their way." White heather stands for good luck. No sight is as lovely as a field of heather in full bloom. In the language of flowers white heather means "good luck."

HELIOTROPE
(Heliotropium peruvianum, H. grandiflorum)
This flower hails from Peru and has been under greenhouse cultivation since 1758. Its odor reminds me of sticky sweet cotton candy. Others claim it smells like cherry pie, honey, or coltsfoot. Heliotrope essence possesses light antiseptic properties.

It falls under the rulership of the sun. Mixed with bay leaves, and tucked under your pillow, it allegedly helps find articles that have been stolen. Heliotrope is said to confer good health, promote tranquility in the home, alleviate arthritis, protect from physical injury, and help make psychic connections with spirits from the Otherworld.

Heliotrope essence is difficult and expensive to extract, so mostly what we see on the market is synthetic. Piesse in *The Art of Perfumery* gives the following heliotrope scent substitute recipe: spiritous extract of vanilla, 1/2 pint, spiritous extract of French rose pomatum 1/4 pint, spiritous extract of orange flower pomatum 2 oz., spiritous extract of ambergris pomatum 1 oz., essential oil of almonds pomatum 5 drops. [16]

The fragrance is said to be favored by those of a Leoine nature; that is, kind and generous, but somewhat authoritarian people. Perhaps because heliotrope always turns toward the sun, it embodies the qualities of "devotion" and "faithfulness" in the language of flowers.

Substitutes for heliotrope include *Allium fragrans*, a rock garden plant, and wild heliotrope (*Euploca convolvulacea*) a native of the Rocky Mountains. Another wild heliotrope, *Phacelia crenulata*, has unpleasantly scented leaves, but heliotrope-like smelling flowers.

HEMLOCK
(Tsuga canadensis)
This evergreen renders an essence produced from the bark that contains a hint of flowers in its piney scent. It makes a delightful addition to woodsy potpourris and American Indian incenses.

HENBANE
(Hyoscyamus niger)
Common Name: Hog's Bean, Devil's-eye
An ingredient of Witches Flying Ointment, it is a dangerous plant that flourishes in wasteground in the Northern hemisphere. In the language of flowers it means "defeat," and "fault." Inhaling the fumes can cause nausea, hallucination, and death. NOT RECOMMENDED.

HONEYSUCKLE
(Lonicera genus)
Common Names: Angel's Breath, Woodbine

This sweetly scented climbing bush is the true woodbine of the Old English herbals. The oil extracted from the flowers resembles lilac. Different scents are emitted by the blooms during the day and at night. The dried blossoms are not recommended for potpourri as they tend to smell decayed.

The essence is touted to possess antibacterial properties and has been proven to kill the staphylococcus bacillus under laboratory conditions.

The perfume is favored by those of an agile, versatile, Gemini nature. Wear when meditating on the nature of non-physical reality and the concept of immortality. Honeysuckle is alleged to sharpen intuition and attract business, fame, love, sex, health and money. It is also associated with eternal love and devotion. This notion originates in the legend of Tristan and Isolde, which states that their love was like the honeysuckle and hazelnut --forever entwined.

HYACINTH
(Hyacinthus orientalis)

This penetratingly sweet fragrance reduces insomnia and draws love and luck. Reputedly it is a compatible male homosexual perfume. Use it as an aid to astral travel by dabbing some on your third eye.

The infelicitous Hyacinthus of Greek mythology was killed accidentally by Apollo during a game of quoits. Out of remorse the god transformed him into a purple hyacinth flower. Perhaps because of this association the flower means "sports," "play" in the language of flower.

IRISH MOSS
(Chondrus crispus)

Known as carrageen after an Irish coastal village where it grows abundantly, this seaweed is chock full of nutrients. During the potato famine many Irish people saved themselves from starvation by eating it. The seaweed is used as a filler in many foods. Today it is harvested off the New England coast. Use Irish moss in Piscean, Lunar, and Earth incenses. The seaweed adds an interesting texture to woodsy or resinous potpourris.

JASMINE
(Jasminum officinale)

Several varieties of the Jupiterian, star-like flower exist, some growing into twenty-foot tall bushes. The original was discovered in Persia, but a yellow Chinese variety (*J. primulinum*) scents tea, another kind has been naturalized in America, and yet another in Europe, where it is trained into trellises.

Approximately 100 species abound. The most expensive, considered the king of love flowers, is grown in Morocco and costs $3,000 per pound, yet does not retain its odor as long as some other kinds.

White jasmine from Grasse, France, is the most frequently used commercially. The highest valued jasmine oil is extracted in the old-fashioned way by *enfleurage*, where the flowers are mixed with purified fat, and the oil rendered is distilled in alcohol. It takes 1,000 pounds of jasmine flowers to yield one pound of oil. Jasmine mingles well with cypress, neroli, rose, and sandalwood. It covers the spectrum of notes from high, to middle and base.

The name in Hindu translates as "moonlight of the grove." Appropriately, in Gem Magic, this flower is associated with the moonstone. To wear this essence assures love, a happy marriage, hope, and happiness. To dream of it means happy news for lovers, good fortune, and an early marriage.

The essential oil or the flowers burned in incense brings good fortune, luck and success, and attracts love. Burn the incense if you want to lift your spirits. In Magic, employ jasmine to charge quartz crystals. The essence is used by aromatherapists to cure impotence and frigidity, and as an antidepressant, cough reliever, and uterine tonic.

The many kinds of jasmine bear different meanings in the language of flowers: Cape jasmine - "transport of joy;" Carolina jasmine - "separation;" Indian jasmine - "I attach myself to you;" Spanish jasmine - "sensibility;" white jasmine - "amiability;" yellow jasmine - "grace, elegance."

Other plants that go by the same name include *Chalcas exotica*, orange jasmine, that smells like oranges and bears a small fruit; *Cestrum nocturnum*, night blooming jasmine, a tropical combination of musk and heliotrope.

JUNIPER
(Juniperus communis)

The berries, wood, and leaves of this hardwood conifer are used in incense-making, potpourris, and perfumes to give an underlying bitter, but invigorating note. The essence, which flavors gin, is obtained by distilling the berries in steam. During the Plague years people burned juniper as a disinfectant and to ward off evil spirits.

Juniper represents "protection" in the language of flowers, perhaps because the bush's low, spreading branches provide shelter for small woodland creatures.

The ancient Greeks burned juniper branches to appease the gods of the Underworld and drive away evil spirits. In rural England, it was long believed that to burn juniper in the hearthfire would protect the home. Similarly, in the Bible the bush hid the baby Christ from Herod's army. In times gone by, pregnant women also burned the branches during childbirth so that the fairies would not spirit away the newborn and leave a changeling in its place.

In herbal medicine and aromatherapy, juniper is reputed as a cure for many ills, including loss of appetite, urinary tract infections, amenorrhea, geriatric diseases, acne, and insomnia. It can be used to clean wounds.

The following recipe for juniper wine comes from *The Practice of Aromatherapy*:

> crushed berries ..... 30 g
> chopped stalks ..... 15 g
> white wine ..... 1 litre
> Leave to steep for four days. Strain and add 30 g sugar.
> sugar.
>
> Take between a liqueur glass and a tumblerful a day (*tonic, aperitif,* diuretic, anticalculous, anti-urinary stones) and indicated for *autumn fevers*. The tonic effect is strengthened with the addition of a pinch of lesser wormwood and 15 g of wild horseradish root.[17]

KAVA-KAVA
(Piper methysticum)
Common Name: Intoxicating Pepper

Add the spicy rhizome of this Hawaiian shrub to love potions and incenses to increase psychic energy. Kava-kava is a narcotic that when emulsified will decrease the pulse rate while increasing the action of the heart, thereby inducing a hypnotic state. It is poisonous in large doses.

LABDANUM
(Cistus ladaniferus)
Common Name: Rock Rose, Cistus
This oleoresin comes from a shrub grown in the Mediterranean. It is used as a fixative in perfumery, and, since it smells something like ambergris, sometimes makes a cheaper substitute. Allegedly wearing this fragrance brings the wearer optimism, audacity in conquering adverse situations, and encourages faithfulness. It is one of the "magnetic" odors in occult perfumery.

LAVENDER
(Lavandula officinalis)
A versatile oil ruled by Mercury, lavender heightens awareness, helps decrease stress, and is a general energizer and stabilizing influence on yin/yang imbalances. Inhale it to help alleviate nasal congestion. The essence destroys typhoid bacillus within 12 hours. Susanne Fischer-Rizzi in *The Complete Aromatherapy Handbook* recommends the following douche to treat vaginal yeast infections. "Combine equal parts of tea tree and lavender oils and use 4 drops of the mixture in 1 pint of rosewater. For added support to the vagina flora, use lactic acid suppositories." [18]

L. vera was introduced to Britain by the Romans. The best quality lavender in the world comes from Norfolk, England. Yardley's is a mixture of lavender, musk, rose absolute, and neroli. French (*L. spica*) and Spanish lavender are inferior, and their plants do not overwinter well. French lavender possesses more strikingly purple flowers, but the fragrance of Spanish lavender is more pungent. If you grow the herb in rich soil, expect fantastic blooms. If you tend the plant in poor soil the blooms will be so-so, but the fragrance will be superior. Lavender grows well from cuttings.

Women in the seventeenth century used to gather in each other's stillrooms just to sniff the pleasant odor of the distillation. Allegedly, the essence helps expel gall stones, and cures muscle pain, skin eruptions, and irritability in infants. Lavender blends well with almost any oil, but be sure to add only a few drops, as it is powerful.

In Magic, lavender invokes Hecate and specifically calls upon her wisdom and circumspection. Lavender flowers accent Isis incense. Anoint an amulet with lavender oil to keep someone from harassing you. The herb means "silent, but fervent love" in the language of flowers. However, the plant also acquired the meaning of "distrust" because Cleopatra's asp was alleged to have secreted itself in a lavender bush. Nonetheless, the tops are burned in offertory and purification rites.

LEMON BALM
(Melissa officinalis)
Common Name: Melissa

This oil is named for the Greek nymph Melissa, or Cybele, who is the bee goddess. This should give you some idea of the number of bees this botanical attracts. A rare and expensive oil distilled in France, it is prized in perfumery. Because it is so expensive many substitutes exist (see LEMONGRASS). In aromatherapy it is an antispasmodic, sedative, and calmative, good for getting rid of migraine headaches.

LEMONGRASS
(Cymbopogon citratus, C. flexuosus)

This grass native to the Indian subcontinent, Jamaica, and the Middle East is an ingredient of Kyphi incense. It was used by the ancient Egyptians in their recipes to enhance their psychic abilities. It is also the oil in the Bible that consecrated Aaron and his son.

The essence's lemony odor is similar to citronella, lemon, melissa, spikenard, and lemon verbena, and makes a reasonable substitute in recipes that call for these scents in perfumery. The fragrance enhances eucalyptus, geranium, juniper, and lime. However, in aromatherapy, each lemony scent carries specific healing characteristics, so substitutions are not appropriate.

Aromatherapists recommend combining lemongrass oil with oregano, thyme, geranium, and vaseline to cure lice. In herbal medicine the essence is ingested to alleviate flatulence and colitis symptoms. Rubbing it on the body helps alleviate the pain of bruises from sports injuries. Otto of lemongrass is also called lemon verbena because it smells somewhat like the verbena plant.

Use it sparingly in citrus and flowery perfumes because the odor is pervasive.

The aroma allegedly chases away fatigue and aids concentration. In Gem Magic, lemongrass is associated with citrine.

LIFE EVERLASTING
(Helicrysum stoechas)

The bright yellow, fuzzy flowers of this everlasting botanical native to Sri Lanka, India and the Moluccas are dried and used in potpourris. They also release an herby aroma when burned.

Another plant which is also called "everlasting", and which is somewhat fragrant and suitable for potpourri is the *Gnaphalium polycephalum* and the *G. ramossissimum*. Of this plant Oliver Wendel Holmes wrote:

> Perhaps the herb everlasting, the fragrant immortelle of our autumn fields, has the most suggestive odour to me of all those that set me dreaming . . . as I inhale the aroma of its pale, dry, rustling flowers. A something it has of sepulchral spicery, as if it had been brought from the core of some great pyramid where it had lain on the breast of a mummified Pharaoh. Something too of immortality in the sad faint sweetness lingering so long in its lifeless petals.[19]

LILAC
(Syringa genus)
Common Names: Duck Bill, Laylock,
Blue Pope Tree, Lily Oak

Most people recognize this May-flowering bush that sometimes grows two stories high. The lilac's odor, while sweet and full-bodied, is faintly spicy, and never cloying. It smells something like tuberose, and used to be a substitute for the more expensive scent. Purple French lilacs emit the strongest fragrance, while white lilacs possess a more delicate aroma. Unfortunately, lilacs loose their smell and turn brown when dried, so they do not flatter potpourris.

Mix three parts lilac oil to one part ginger flower oil, and anoint your breasts to arouse passion. Folk superstition recommends anointing with lilac essence as protection from vampires! It is a Jupiterian and Mercurian fragrance, and can be used in spells for wealth and increase. Add some to a light bulb scent ring in your young child's room to help foment mental development.

LILY
(Lilium genus)

Louise Beebe Wilder finds the scent of the Libra-governed lily "languorous and decadent," [20] but I love its warm fragrance borne on the gentle springtime breezes. For me, lilies represent rebirth and faith in miracles. Ancient Greeks consecrated this flower to their goddess Hera. The Egyptians manufactured a strong perfume to treat female complaints from the lily. In times gone by, it was believed that lilies represented all that was celibate, cosmic, and pure, and that the plague would not enter the house where the lily grew. In the language of flowers, lily represents "majesty," perhaps because its regal bloom stands head and shoulders above all other Spring flowers. On the Tree of Life the Madonna lily is associated with Binah.

Not all lilies smell sweet—some have a musty odor, others are downright unpleasant, and still others, including most day lilies, do not emit any fragrance at all.

LILY-OF-THE-VALLEY
(Convallaria majalis)

This delicate flower thrives in the shadows of damp woodlands and mountain valleys. Similarly scented botanicals include *Pyrola rotundifolia*, a rock garden plant and Pipsissewa (*Chimaphila umbellata*), a creeping evergreen common throughout the United States. If you grow lily-of-the-valley, keep it away from children and animals, as it is poisonous. Also, since in perfumery its penetrating sweetness does not blend well with lilac yet blooms around the same time, I suggest you not plant them together in your garden. This is an expensive scent because it is difficult to extract from the flower. Blend the essence into skin beautifying formulas. The fragrance combines well with cinnamon, jasmine, rose, orange, tuberose, and oakmoss.

The May-blooming flower that celebrates the Springtime, symbolizes "return of happiness" in the language of flowers. It is also known as Nuit Oil, and invokes the Egyptian goddess of the night. The chaste, white flowers often appear in paintings of the Virgin Mary because they signify purity. The plant once was called

Our Lady's-tears. Medieval monks named the plant "ladder-to-heaven" because of the step-like arrangement of the flowers on the stem. In Irish legend the Little People ran up and down the flower ladders and rang the blossoms like bells. Lily-of-the-valley on a light bulb ring in the bedroom promotes a restful night's sleep.

LINDEN
(Tilia genus)

This stately tree also known as the lime tree, attracts myriads of bees to its ambrosial blossoms in July. Bathe your face in linden flower tea to smooth the skin.

Linden symbolizes "conjugal love" in the language of flowers. In Greek legend Zeus, travelling across the land of Phrygia, was hospitably received by a faithful old couple. In return they asked that when it came their time they might die together. Zeus granted their wish, and at the moment of their deaths transformed the husband into an oak and the wife into a linden.

LOTUS
(Nelumbium genus, Nymphaea alba)
White Pond Lily

The tangy undertones of this intoxicatingly scented flower makes it an interesting addition to many perfume blends. The fragrance of the blossom is enhanced after dark.

Lotus is sacred to the Chinese, Tibetans, East Indians, and Egyptians because it symbolizes the supremacy of mind over matter. Anoint yourself with the essence to fortify yourself and keep your spiritual strength safe from harm and depletion. Burn lotus oil in incense to ease emotional pain, lengthen your lifespan, and energize yourself. Use it in rituals to fulfill seemingly impossible dreams. It increases fertility and allegedly makes a woman irresistible to a man. In the language of flowers, lotus means "eloquence." In Christian mythology it is a symbol of chastity.

MAGNOLIA
(Magnolia genus)

Magnolia trees can reach up to 70 feet in height. The languorously scented perfume allegedly facilitates psychic development and meditation and helps locate items that have been lost. The fragrance combines well with orange blossom, almond, rose, tuberose, and violet. It is said to be worn by those of an argumentative nature. The perfume is sometimes used in love spells. Sprinkle it on the bed sheets to ignite passionate love.

MARIGOLD
(Calendula officinalis)
Common Names: Pot Marigold, English Marigold

This merry, golden flower is grown as a perennial in Mediterranean climates. The Latin name originates in a word that means "the first of the month," as the flower seems to come into bloom at that time around the Mediterranean. Marigold petals brighten potpourris.

Burn the petals in incense, or anoint your temples with the pungent oil to make fairies visible. Use tincture of marigold in money-draw oils, or add dried flowers sparingly to prosperity incenses.

During Medieval times, a combination of marigold, sage and rue juice was believed to keep away the plague. Nowadays, a marigold infusion is sometimes used as a yellow hair or cloth dye, and as a substitute for tumeric in cooking. In aromatherapy, it is consumed to strengthen the heart and liver, eliminate toxins, and rid the psyche of sorrow.

By tradition, this flower protects and blesses the departed soul, and causes a person to feel merry. In the Orient, the flower is said to soothe grief, but in the language of flowers, it means "grief," "pain," and "chagrin." In Victorian times, a person wore a marigold in the hair to mean "sorrow of the mind," on the breast to signify "boredom," and over the heart to symbolize "pangs of love."

A few petals added to your daily bath will cause others to respect and admire you.

MASTIC
(Pistacia lentiscus, P. atlantica)

A gum resin mainly produced in Lebanon, it is difficult to obtain in this country due to perennial upheavals in the Middle East. Sometimes it can be found as a varnish ingredient in artists' supplies stores at exorbitant prices. The fragrance released by burning mastic is heavenly--both sharp and light at the same time. It combines well with honeysuckle, lavender, mimosa, and sweet pea. It is an ingredient of Turkish liqueur, and is sometimes used in breath sweeteners.

Mastic is ruled by Mercury and is the key component of Merlin's Magic incense. In the tarot, this scent is associated with the Magician. Add it to divination incenses along with cinnamon, juniper, patchouli, and sandalwood. The fragrance helps stimulate the mind.

MIGNONETTE
(Reseda odorata)

In previous centuries, the exquisite fragrance of mignonette permeated the streets of London because it was an ubiquitous window box plant. In spite of the less than showy blooms and tendency to spread like a weed, its charming bouquet made this botanical so popular that it was christened in English with a French name that means "little darling." In the language of flowers it came to mean "your qualities surpass your charms!" Unfortunately, the scent is not much used in perfumery because it is difficult to separate the fragrance from the plant without altering its characteristics.

Recently I obtained mignonette seeds mail order from Nichol's Garden Nursery, planted them in the two tubs that flank my front steps, and by summer was rewarded with a heavenly fragrance. I offset the plant's scraggly appearance by interplanting more showy, taller, but fragrance-free annuals and perennial bulbs. The oil is thought to bring harmony to the environment.

MIMOSA
(Acacia genus, A. floribunda)
Common Name: Tassel Tree

This yellow-colored, saucy prophesying oil also exudes honey-like undertones. Anoint your third eye with it before retiring to encourage psychic dreams and calm the spirit. In aromatherapy the essential oil is used as a tonic for the liver and gallbladder.

MISTLETOE
(Viscum album, Phorandendron flavescens)
American Mistletoe

Mistletoe is a parasite that grows on the poplar, hawthorne, willow, and less frequently, the oak. Modern Medicine considers it poisonous to ingest. Nonetheless, it was employed by the Druids in Magic in order to see beyond the cycle of rebirth. The Druids also thought that the plant cured sterility and epilepsy, and protected against sorcerers.

In Norse myth, the lowly mistletoe inadvertently caused the death of Balder the Beautiful, beloved son of Odin and Freya.

Mistletoe is a famous aphrodisiac and element in love divinations. Wear the perfume at your temples, throat, and ankles to keep away negativity. Add it to floor wash to attract patrons to a business. In the language of flowers this botanical means "I surmount all obstacles."

MOUNTAIN ASH
(Sorbus aucaparia, S. americana)
Common Names: Rowan, Quickbeam

The bright, orange berries of this tree, if carefully dried so they do not shrivel, are gaily decorative in potpourri. Spread mountain ash leaves at the Quarters during the Beltane ceremony. It is said that if you plant a rowan tree next to your house lightning will never strike. My house is flanked by two mountain ash trees, and we've not been struck by lightning yet, so obviously it must be true(!)

MUGWORT
(Artemisia vulgaris)
Common Names: Felon Herb, St. John's Herb

The Latin name shows that this plant was once associated with the goddess Artemis. The lowly, common artemisia is used in scrying incense and to stuff dream pillows. Layer some in your shoes to keep alert. In Pagan times, mugwort was known as the "mother of herbs" because it was believed to hold the power to drive off imps and devils.

More practically, mugwort is a Chinese remedy for rheumatism, and was used to flavor beer, and as a condiment to cut the greasy taste of poultry and beef. In aromatherapy, it is a strong emmenagogue, antispasmodic, cholagogue, and vermifuge.

The dried leaves hold up well in everlasting bouquets, and lend a brownish to silvery color and feathery texture to wreaths.

MUSK
(Moschus moschiferus)

This potent scent, which allegedly appeals to the deepest levels of the psyche, is retained by almost any material, including polished steel! The mortar in many mosques is permeated with the fragrance.

The highest valued musk is extracted from the glandular sack of the Himalayan musk deer, also found in China, Korea, Tibet, and Siberia. Please do not buy it, as its popularity is forcing the musk deer to be hunted to extinction, this in spite of the fact that there is a hole in the deer's skin through which the walnut-sized gland can be easily extracted without harming the animal. Although over 80 synthetic musks exist, two basic aromas--dark, and light are used in perfumery, and they are quite distinct. This scent is associated with Chokmah on the Tree of Life.

Musk is a famed Arabian love oil. Rub it on your hands and feet to instill yourself with self-assuredness. Apply it to your third eye during meditation to open your chakras to divine wisdom. The synthetic oil and crystals are burned in love incenses to draw affection and prosperity.

Musk ambrette seed (*Hibiscus abelmoschus*) from the musk mallow can be ground and used as a substitute for musk in incense making. A California musk plant (*Mimulus moschatus*), which grows alongside streams in the West, can also be used.

MYRRH
(Commiphora myrrha)

This gum resin from a tree native to the Middle East and North Africa is an antiseptic, astringent, emmenagogue, expectorant, stimulant, tonic, and superior gum and throat wash. It is effective against indigestion, flatulence and uterine and pulmonary hemorrhages. In aromatherapy, frankincense has superseded myrrh in popularity in our time.

Myrrh is a fixative in perfumery and potpourri, and evens out Oriental blends. The smokey, mysterious, woodsy resin forms an essential part of many incenses, including Mystic Veil, Isis, and Persephone. In many ancient religions the resin was burned in temples to guard against evil.

The bush is a Christian symbol of continence. In Greek legend, the infant Adonis was born from a myrrh tree. Along with frankincense, myrrh was burned in liturgical rites throughout the ancient world, and was an Egyptian embalming ingredient. The oil was burned in ritual lamps and temples. Hebrew women used to purify themselves with it.

Magically, the resin is employed in rites of exorcism and Saturn, to drive and bind spells, and to attract love and success. It is associated with the sun, Jupiter, Saturn, Aries, and Aquarius. Spraying a cologne mixture of myrrh and rosewater throughout your loved one's home and wardrobe is alleged to seal the courtship.

MYRTLE
(Myrtus communis)
Common Name: Bayberry Bark

The dark green, leathery evergreen leaves when burned release a clean scent, similar to eucalyptus, but more spicy than medicinal. Myrtle blends well with bergamot, clove, cypress, sage, lavender, lily, orange blossom, and rosemary. Do not confuse this tree with the creeping botanical also known as myrtle or periwinkle, *Vinca major* and *V. minor*.

Myrtle incense invokes Aphrodite/Venus. It is also said to help preserve youth. The temple dedicated to this goddess in ancient Rome was surrounded by a myrtle grove. Romans wore myrtle wreaths at April marriage ceremonies. In Greece the botanical was fashioned into wreaths as burial crowns for the dead. In the language of flowers, myrtle signifies "love." During the nineteenth century myrtle flower water was popular in France. Fischer-Rizzi claims that essential oil of myrtle helps balance people with addictions, low self-esteem, and self-destructive tendencies by showing them their inner beauty and preparing them for better times. She also says that the aroma may help the dying accept their fate and gain higher wisdom. [21]

By tradition, to dream of myrtle presages many lovers and a legacy. If you are married, it foretells a second marriage, many children, wealth, and life to a ripe old age.

The leaves of *Myrica cerifera*, also known as myrtle or candleberry, render a more tangy, Christmasy fragrance that is rumored to attract money when sprinkled each week in a billfold or on the threshold of a business. *M. californica*, also known as wax myrtle, also possesses very aromatic leaves.

Recipe for Portugal Essence
1 part orange flower water
1 part rosewater
1/2 part myrtle water
28 drops musk
28 drops ambergris

NARCISSUS
(Narcissus genus)

Narcissus fragrances vary from pear-like to magnolia-like, but in general, the odor is considered intoxicating. The color of the petals are pale white or yellow, the yellow possessing the faintest scent.

In Greek myth the dizzying aroma of the flower was considered fatal, as the nymphs had built a funeral pyre with it for the god, Narcissus. Persephone was gathering the flower when Hades snatched her up and carried her off to the Underworld. The ancient Egyptians fashioned funeral wreaths from the blossoms. Contrastingly, the flower is also sacred to the Fates because the narcissus is a harbinger of Spring, portending rebirth, new beginnings, and hope.

The tantalizing, floral perfume is alleged to heighten self-esteem (it is related to the word "narcissism"), and brings peace, enlightenment, patience, affection, harmony, a pleasant sleep, and Virgoan vibrations. In the tarot, the fragrance is associated with the Hierophant trump. Burn narcissus oil in incense to rekindle the sexual excitement of a dragging love affair.

NARCISSE is a synthetic oil that possesses a distinctive scent reminiscent of vetiver. Use it in Compelling perfume.

NUTMEG
(Myristica fragrans)

This peppery aromatic from a tree native to Java, Indonesia, and the West Indies lends a spicy note to blends. Nutmeg of India (mace) is the whole nut, and is prized in Magic as a botanical for mojo bags to bring love and money.

OAKMOSS
(Evernia prunastri)

Oakmoss lichen, popular in potpourri, is a resinoid in perfumes because it combines well with many scents including patchouly, tonka bean, vanilla, vetivert, all florals, and also accentuates the freshness of citrus blends. Among its virtues is its fixative property. The web-like, feathery, gray color lends a subtle, woodsy note to potpourri. Uncut oakmoss is used to make the skirt and body of Cajun Witch dolls. It is another occult power oil, useful when invoking the elementals.

OLIVE
(Olea europaea)

Pure, rectified olive oil provides an excellent base in which to distill other essences, as it is sacred to Minerva, goddess of wisdom. It is available at most pharmacies under the name "sweet oil." This oil possesses antidiabetic qualities and carries no odor.

OPOPANAX

The root and stem of this plant, native to Southern Europe, Somalia, and Persia, exudes a dark, bittersweet resin that when hardened, is used as a fixative in incenses and perfumery. It is probably the same scent that is called myrrh in the Bible. It is associated with Pluto.

ORANGE BLOSSOM
(Citrus aurantium, C. bigarradia)
bitter orange - superior quality,
(C. sinesis)
Sweet Orange, Portugal Orange - inferior quality
Common Names: Neroli, Bigarrade

Orange blossom oil is steam-distilled from the flowers of bitter orange trees grown in the United States, France, Morocco, Egypt, Tunisia, and Sicily. The blossoms are gathered by hand. It takes one ton of flowers to produce one quart of oil, which is antiseptic and lightly hypnotic. Essence of bitter orange (C. bergamia - see BERGAMOT) is extracted from the peel.

In Greek legend, one of Zeus's marriage gifts to Hera was an orange. Brides still wear orange blossoms on their wedding day to insure a long, happy marriage. In the language of flowers, orange blossoms stand for "chastity." Orange blossom is associated with Uranus, and in Gem Magic with the diamond.

This subtle, mysterious, inviting essence mingles well with bergamot, cedar, geranium, linalool, orange, rose, rosemary, and sandalwood. Add the flowers to love incenses.

A once popular perfume, Portugal Essence, (see recipe above under MYRTLE) is derived in part from the peel of the sweet orange tree. Sweet orange oil rounds out almost any perfume, and adds warmth to spicy blends. It is a favorite oil of children. In Health Magic, orange blossom oil counteracts depression, insomnia, PMS, hysteria, colitis, and psychosomatic illnesses, and moistens and deodorizes skin.

An old recipe for Fairy Butter is found in *The Receipt Book of Elizabeth Clelands*, published in 1759:

> Take the Yolks of four hard Eggs, and half a Pound of Loaf Sugar beat and sifted, a Pound Butter; bray them in a clean Bowl with two spoonfuls of Orange-flower Water; when it is well mixed, force it through the corner of a thin Canvas Strainer in little Heaps on a Plate. It is a very pretty Supper Dish.[22]

The peel makes a spicy addition to Mercurian incense. The burning of the peel releases the essential oil. Save your orange, lemon, and tangerine peels, scrape off the white part, cut them into small pieces, and dry them in shallow trays in the sunshine. Add to potpourris.

ORCHID
(Orchidaceae)

Even though we usually associate them with the tropics, orchids actually grow in a bewildering variety of colors and scents in almost all regions of the world. For instance, *Calypso borealis*, named for the nymph of the north, grows in cold, mountainous regions. The *Habenaria albida*, the Newfoundland orchid, flourishes there and smells like vanilla.

Some orchids exude different aromas during the day than at night. In general, all orchid fragrances allegedly help focus complete concentration on the task at hand and promote creativity.

Orchids belong to the zodiac sign, Libra, and also to the planet Mercury.

ORRIS
(Iris germanica, var. florentina)
This is the root of a kind of iris also known as yellow flag, that is grown in Southern Europe. Both *I. germanica* and *I. pallida* are used in perfumery, but the Florentine variety is considered the most fragrant. It makes a fine fixative, especially for potpourris. It blends well with violet because it smells like this flower, as well as with other floral scents and lavender. Employ orris in love charms. The sachet is known as Queen Elizabeth Love Powder, and is applied to the body with a powder puff to attract and fascinate a lover. It also is reputed to enhance creativity.

From a related plant, the May flowering common garden iris, is extracted a sweet and light essence used to scent soaps and cosmetic creams. This iris falls under the rulership of Libra and is sacred to Hera.

PALMAROSA
(Cymbopogon martini)
Palmarosa oil smells something like roses and is often used to adulterate this expensive essence. However, it possesses its own virtues and is used in cosmetics to help banish wrinkles and pimples. It also is a versatile blender that mixes successfully with almost any other oil.

PANSY
(Viola tricolor)
In Shakespeare's time it was believed that the warmly fragrant juice from pansies would cause others to fall madly in love with the wearer. In another legend the flower is said to calm the emotions.

Although violas fall under the dominion of Saturn, they are sacred to St. Valentine, and are used in love talismans. Add pansies to love incenses, and spread some in your shoes to attract the perfect mate.

PASSION FLOWER
(Passiflora caerulea)
Common Name: Maypops

The refined essence extracted from the white and purple flowers of this climbing vine is alleged to make the indifferent lover burn with passion. The scent combines well with herby flowers like thyme and rosemary, as well as violet. When inhaled, the fragrance is alleged to calm the savage breast.

The plant is associated with the Passion of Christ; hence its name, and perhaps is one of the reasons why in occult perfumery the fragrance is used for blessing and prayer. The tendrils are symbolic of the cords that bound Jesus on the cross; the three stigma are like the nails with which Christ was hung on the Cross; the leaves resemble the thirty pieces of silver for which He was betrayed; the bud represents the Eucharist; the half-open flowers, the Star of the East; the five purple slashes on the corona, the Crown of Thorns; the five stamens, the Five Wounds; finally the ten petals, the Ten Apostles minus Peter and Judas.

This botanical represents "belief," "susceptibility," and "superstition" in the language of flowers. It is used as a blessing oil.

PATCHOULY
(Pogostemon patchouli)

A definitely yang scent, but lacking in the burning sensation usually associated with these oils, patchouly exudes a dark, persistent, musky, mossy, offbeat odor. Patchouly is the product of the leaves and stems of a mint-like shrub grown in Java, India, and Singapore. It combines well with heady aromas like jasmine, labdanum, Oriental blends, sandalwood, musk, tonka, ylang-ylang and white rose. East Indian and Singapore are the most common varieties.

Formerly patchouly was used to scent shawls and linens in India in order to drive away moths. By analogy in Magic, it banishes foes, especially on the astral plane, and breaks off love affairs. Yet patchouly also brings peace and contentment to the home. It is an ingredient of some love oils. Patchouly leaves are a component of Graveyard Dust. The earthy redolence in incense draws money and the power of the Gnomes.

This fixative with an extremely low evaporation rate heals wounds and tightens sagging skin. The essential oil helps cure vaginal yeast infections. India ink is permeated with patchouly and camphor.

PEONY
(Paeonia genus)

In *The Fragrant Garden*, Louise Beebe Wilder describes the fragrance of peony:

> At their best, they may be said to have a coarse Rose scent. In it is much of the sweetness and transparency of Rose perfume, much of its refreshing quality, but back of this is something undefinable that is a little rank, a suggestion of something medicinal perhaps...This curious sub-odor, so to speak, is most marked in the single and semi-double varieties, and it is said to be due to the strong, rather rank odour of the pollen that predominates over what little scent the petals may possess.[23]

She goes on to say that in her opinion, the pale pink variety smells best.

The pink to dark red flower petals brighten potpourris. The oil extracted from the flower keeps the devil away and dispels negativity. Witches consider it a perfume of good fortune and a scent that facilitates meditation and psychic self-development. It means "shame" in the language of flowers because the large blossoms were fancied to conceal guilty Nymphs!

PEPPER
(Piper genus)

Black pepper originates from green berries, while white pepper is taken from mature, red berries. In small doses the pungent odor combines well with sandalwood and frankincense. Use it in spells to cause an enemy to flee. Pepper also adds piquancy to a relationship.

PEPPERMINT
(Mentha piperita)

Pluto is said to have changed his wife's rival Mentha into a peppermint plant; so in the language of flowers this herb refers to both the coldness of fear and the warmth of love.

In *The Practice of Aromatherapy*, Jean Valnet claims that peppermint tea may cause insomnia. Perhaps this is part of the basis for why some psychics drink it at bedtime to "dream true;" that is, produce prophetic dreams. Certainly peppermint is a refreshing scent that clears the mind and calms the nerves.

Peppermint essence, extracted by steam distillation, kills staphylococcus and neutralizes the tuberculosis bacillus; so this may be used in aromatherapy to help cure these diseases. Peppermint also possesses carminative, antispasmodic, and antiseptic properties. It is a valuable remedy for dizziness, nausea, and morning sickness.

By tradition, the odor drives away enemies and is hexing agent. The scent is said to bring balance and justice into one's life. It is associated with ecology, partnership, the laws of Karma, and justice. It also draws love and excitement into one's life. In the language of flowers, peppermint symbolizes cordiality. Add a drop of this activating oil to other fragrances in order to set their influences into motion.

Other mints besides peppermint common as potpourri ingredients include spearmint, curly mint, orangemint, bergamot, and wintergreen.

PETTIGRAIN
(See ORANGE BLOSSOM for genus name)

The fragrance, derived from the small branches and leaves of the bitter orange, is alleged to sharpen awareness and energize the mind. It combines well with neroli, bergamot, and Oriental-style perfumes. Pettigrain has a sharp fragrance quite distinct from the peppery scent of bergamot or the bright, flowery fragrance of orange blossom. It is used widely in perfumery.

PIKAKI

This is the Hawaiian wedding flower that confers the blessings of love and union on those who wear it. It blends well with ginger blossom.

PINE

(Pinus genus*)*

The essential oil of this evergreen tree native to the cooler regions of the world is obtained by a steam distillation of the needles. In aromatherapy and herbal medicine, the essence is used to cure genito-urinary tract infections, flu, and impotence. A few drops in a facial cleanser makes an invigorating rubefacient. Add four to six drops of the essential oil to a cupful of honey water and drink several times a day to alleviate flu symptoms.

An oil sacred to Poseidon, pine is said to repel evil and cleanse the aura of negativity. After anointing yourself with it at the new moon, you can begin anew with a fresh, courageous heart.

The resin, collected from wounds on the trunk of the tree, bark, and needles, are essential ingredients in many incenses, including those that invoke American Indian and forest spirits. Inhaling the smoke from burning pine resin and needles brings strength, fortitude, and peace of mind.

PINEAPPLE

(Ananas comosus A sativus)

The British Victorians admired this fragrant plant for its scent, and also because it was so difficult for them to cultivate in their cold climate. In the language of flowers, pineapple stands for "perfection."

The fragrance is thought to bring back a departed lover: at the full moon, anoint an orange-colored candle with the perfume for a male, or a pink candle, for a female, and burn for fifteen minutes each day until the candle is extinguished or until the moon changes phase. Add the perfume to incense to lift your spirits and purify and protect you.

The bromelin enzyme which is plentiful in pineapple, breaks down protein; so can be used as a digestive aid.

POPPY
(Papaver rhoeas)

The red poppy is a long time symbol of fallen warriors. The Greeks dedicated the flower to Demeter and Artemis. This flower is also an analgesic and sedative in herbal medicine. The colorful blossoms tint wine and tea, and make lovely additions to potpourri. This is not *P. somniferum*, the opium poppy.

The scent is alleged to draw large amounts of money fast. Inhale smoke from the incense fumes to divine the future. Poppy seeds (90,000 are contained in one pound!) are an ingredient of Psychic Vision incense. On the Tree of Life poppies are associated with Malkuth.

Anna Riva suggests the following divination spell in *The Modern Herbal Spellbook:* "To divine the future, fling a few seeds under burning coals with a question in mind. If the smoke rises lightly and disappears quickly, it is fortunate. If the smoke hangs heavy and low, it is certainly a bad omen." [24]

PRICKLY ASH
(Zanthoxylum clavus)

The flowers, leaves, and fruits of this thorny tree are extremely sweet, and suitable for incense and potpourri. The berries can be pulverized and used in love incenses and in formulas to draw a potential spouse.

PRIMROSE
(Primula genus, *Enothera biennis)*

Sacred to Freya, this oil attracts love. It also allegedly extracts the truth from liars. The flower symbolizes "early youth" in the language of flowers, and so is a perfect scent to wear at the New Year. Many of the finer scented primroses are native to China.

Oil of Evening Primrose (*Enothera biennis*), recently has been touted as a skin and body rejuvenator. Contrary to its name, only some species of the plant flower at night. The oil is pearly and light, reminiscent of orange flowers and jasmine.

QUASSIA

(Picrasma excelsa)
Native to Jamaica
(Quassia amara)
Native to Panama, Venezuela, and Brazil

This ash-like tree, also known as bitter wood, bears clusters of rosy flowers, and grows from fifty to one hundred feet high. The bark is used medicinally, in incense, and is a safe pesticide (make a tea and spray it on plants). It also kills moths and flies. Formerly brewers sometimes substituted quassia for hops. It is a bitter stomachic, antispasmodic in cases of fever, vermicide, and slight narcotic. Quassia increases the appetite when ingested in small doses with ginger as an infusion.

Quassia chips burned in love incense restore harmony in love relationships.

ROSE

(Rosa genus)

Queen of fragrances, and meaning "love" and "beauty" in the language of flowers, the rose is decidedly a feminine scent, often associated with love and secrecy. It has been a favorite scent in all ages, but was especially liked by the Romans:

When Nero honored the house of a Roman noble with his imperial presence at dinner, there was something more than flowers; the host was put to an enormous expense by having (according to royal custom) all his fountains flinging up rose-water. While the jets were pouring out the fragrant liquid, while rose-leaves were on the ground, in the cushions on which the guests lay, hanging in garlands on their brows and in wreaths around their necks, the *couleur de rose* pervaded the dinner itself, and a rose pudding challenged the appetites of the guests. To encourage digestion there was rose-wine, which Heliogabalus was not only simple enough to drink, but extravagant enough to bathe in. He went even further, by having the public swimming-baths filled with wine of roses and absinth.[25]

Kinds and qualities of rose oil abound, depending on the type of petals used. Most of what is sold is synthetic because it takes 5 tons of petals to produce 1 pound of essence by steam distillation. Obviously this makes the price of the otto prohibitively expensive in most cases. Some highly scented varieties include: French rose (*Rosa gallica*—only lightly scented as an oil, but the fragrance of the petals increases as they are dried); pride of the graces, cabbage rose or Provencale rose (*Rosa centifolia*); dog rose (*R. canina*); wild briar rose (*Rosa rugosa*—the sturdiest); damask rose (*R. damascena*—which in the language of flowers refers to a "brilliant complexion" and "beauty ever new," the source of much rosewater and attar of rose).

Tea roses carry a more spicy, musty scent because they retain a strain of the old musk rose. Other exotically perfumed roses include: field rose (*R. arvensis*, which smells like mignonette); *R. cathayensis* (which is an especially fragrant climbing variety); cinnamon rose (*R. cinnamomea*—guess what this smells like !); Cherokee rose (*R. laevigata*—reminiscent of gardenia); musk rose (*R. moschata*—not surprisingly redolent of musk).

Usually the smaller, dustier looking blooms are more highly scented than the showy blossoms bred for looks rather than scent. Red roses are usually more intensely scented than the white or yellow varieties.

When collecting petals for fragrance, the ideal time is at sunrise, just before the petals begin to open.

Bulgarian rose otto, the most expensive oil, distills the essence from thirty roses to produce one drop. In ancient Greece, rose oil was the supreme offering to Aphrodite, from whose blood the rose is said to have sprung. It is an all-purpose anointing oil for altar cloths, candles, sacred objects, tools, and even acolytes!

It possesses the added virtue of being slightly antiseptic as well, and is good for conjunctivitis and migraine headaches. Rose oil is thought to neutralize anger and bring peace and harmony.

In occult perfumery, rose is associated with secrecy, the activities of the vegetative life of humankind, and rose quartz. Mellie Uyldert in *The Psychic Garden* claims that roses are for those who are prepared to suffer for their happiness, who embrace life in its fullness here and now, and who live on earth with the knowledge of God in their hearts. [26]

Use small amounts of the petals and buds in incense to add appropriate color and to invoke Isis, attract love and passion, and increase your personal magnetism. When burned, the petals smell like burning leaves, so use sparingly!

ROSEMARY
(Rosmarinus officinalis)

The name which means "sea dew" refers to the fact that this pot plant herb with dark green, spiky, fragrant leaves flourishes best near the sea. Sailors can smell its refreshing, resinous odor twenty miles from land. Naturally, rosemary makes a pleasant home air purifier. Although surprisingly not indigenous to Britain, it has been naturalized there since ancient times, and has come to be known as one of the primary English occult herbs.

The odor is strongly medicinal, but refreshing smelling, aptly named in the language of flowers as "your presence revives me." Rosemary forms the basis of the famous Hungary Water, which allegedly turned a seventy-year-old princess into a sexy, seductive lass of seventeen, and prompted the King of Poland to ask for her hand in marriage. The oil is believed to bring serenity and wisdom, prevent a thief from stealing, attract good ghosts and repel evil ones, discourage nightmares, unhex a person, preserve youth, and improve the memory. In ancient Greece, students wore rosemary sprigs in their hair to help them remember their lessons. Along with verbena, geranium, and thyme, it is an ingredient of Holy Water.

The needles exude a crisp aroma when burned in incense. Rosemary is an ingredient of many Celtic recipes because it was one of the few incense-making plants that could be grown in Britain. The scent blends well with spices, frankincense, lavender, and rose.

In aromatherapy, oil of rosemary is said to work as a heart tonic and cure for fainting spells, migraine headaches, jaundice, and impotence. Drink 3 or 4 drops of the essence three times a day in honey water. Ancient Roman bakers believed that bread baked on a bed of rosemary could cure a person of dizziness and restore the sense of smell.

ROSEWOOD
(Aniba roseadora)

The distillation of the wood, grown in Brazil, is woodsy-rosy sweet, and makes a solid middle note blender in perfumery. If you are able to find the powdered wood, it forms a fine incense base.

RUE
(Ruta graveolens)
Common Name: Herb of Grace

Rue is grown in the temperate regions of the world. It is called herb of grace because rue branches formerly were used in the Roman Catholic Church to sprinkle Holy Water before Mass. In England sprigs of rue used to be placed in the bar of the Central Criminal Court to protect the judge, jury, and lawyers from infections spread by prisoners who were confined in unsanitary conditions.

During the Middle Ages, the strong smell of rue was believed to drive away plague, fleas, and lice. Rue is an antispasmodic and helps destroy intestinal worms.

Add small amounts to incense for protection and to guard against Black Magic, or to renew your life.

SAFFRON
(Crocus sativus)

This is an expensive ingredient harvested from the stigma of the *Crocus sativus* (4,000 flowers are needed to make one ounce). It is a favorite in devotional, solar, and Jupiterian incenses. Saffron burned in incense helps bring success to all undertakings and increases self-confidence, independence, leadership, enthusiasm, and clairvoyance. The botanical symbolizes the philosopher king in all his magnificence, dynamism, and wisdom.

If you cannot afford the high price, substitute dried marigold or safflower petals (*Carthamus tinctoria*—Mexican saffron). The yellow flower petals also make a bright addition to potpourris.

Bake it into crescent-shaped cookies as the Phoenicians did, to honor their goddess, Ashtoreth. In the language of flowers, saffron warns against abuse or overindulgence. The flower earned this reputation because it used to be taken in alcoholic infusions.

SAGE
(Salvia officinalis)

Dry the gray leaves of this versatile culinary herb to add an herby aroma to incense. Wild mountain sage is best. *S. sclarea* (see CLARY SAGE) is the variety used in aromatherapy and perfumery. The Chinese so valued this herb as a tea that at one time they traded to the Dutch their own black tea for it pound for pound. It is said that sage prevents aging, and confers wisdom. It is alleged to thrive or wither in the garden according to the fortunes of the owner.

Pineapple sage (*S. rutilans*) smells like pineapple and grows like a low bush with cream and green leaves. I have found it to be a great plant in my rock garden, that thrives in spite of the dry, windy climate and sometimes shocking neglect.

Sage brush (*Artemisia tridentata*), a highly aromatic artemisia common to the high plains and deserts of the West, smells like a meadow after a summer shower.

Sage was a well-known panacea from early times, and was called "sacred herb" by the Romans. Among its numerous uses, it is a diuretic, antiseptic, stimulant, and promoter of conception. Aromatherapists claim that if you apply sage or rosemary to your skin it will regulate the capillary action, and revitalize it. Do not ingest the essential oil because its method of distillation makes it toxic.

SAINT JOHN'S WORT
(Hypericum perforatum)
Common Name: Rosin Rose

Gather this yellow-flowered, woody perennial herb at the Summer Solstice and throw it in the Needfire. It sharpens psychic abilities and increases fertility. The Greeks believed its fragrance chased away evil spirits; similarly, the Roman Catholic Church uses it in exorcisms. Do not ingest, as it is poisonous and can cause skin burns. Together with lavender the essential oil of St. John's wort helps alleviate earaches.

SALTPETER

This ingredient of quick-lighting coals enables them to fire up rapidly, and can be added to incenses for the same purpose. Unfortunately, saltpeter has a somewhat acrid odor when burned, which may mar the subtlety of accompanying scents. Since this substance is ruled by Mars, if you add saltpeter to incense, it links the product to this influence. I advise you use saltpeter only in Mars and Saturn blends, or when the purpose of the ritual calls for it. (For more on quick-lighting coals, see chapter 4.)

SANDALWOOD
(Santalum album)

This familiar oil is extracted from the inner bark of a parasitic tree that grows to thirty feet in East India, China, the West Indies, and Australia. The sandalwood with which the Hindus built their temples is the brown variety. The highest quality sandalwood is known as mysore. As of this writing, sandalwood is becoming scarce on the market because India is refusing to export it. A reasonable substitute, if anyone cares to grow and harvest it, is the *Myoporum sandwicense*, the so-called "bastard sandalwood tree." It smells very much like the real McCoy.

Santal (*Pterocarpus santalibus*—a related wood) is red; the smell is woodsy and spicy, and it combines well with jasmine, rose, neroli, verbena, vetivert, ylang-ylang, and benzoin.

Medicinally, sandalwood successfully treats acne and genito-urinary tract infections, prostate trouble, and sinusitis, although it is somewhat poisonous. It also acts as an expectorant and antispasmodic.

Anoint Ouija boards, pendulums, and tarot cards with the perfume to bring fast, accurate answers. Dab the oil on your third eye when performing past life recall. The fragrance is said to draw beneficial healing vibrations and promote spirituality. At the New Year, Burmese women take to the streets and sprinkle passersby with rose and sandalwood water to wash away the sins of the old year.

The bark, either in small pieces, or pulverized, is employed in incense-making. Burn it to aid concentration. It is a popular ingredient in Oriental blends, and is a prized dry-spicy-woodsy fixative and blender in many perfumes, often comprising as much as 50% of the blend. The fragrance harmonizes well with the other woody scents, spices, frankincense, and lavender, and especially those fragrances that help make men more attractive to women.

SASSAFRAS
(Sassafras albidum)
Common Name: Cinnamonwood

You may remember the aroma from childhood, because sassafras was an ingredient of old-fashioned American candy. The FDA now considers it unsafe to ingest because one of its chemical constituents is a potential carcinogen. As of this writing, it is easily obtainable for incense and herbal teas from health food stores. Burn the bark to add a sweet fragrance to your incenses.

SEA LAVENDER
(Limonium carolinianum, Statice latifolia)
The dainty fragrance emitted by this plant that grows wild in American sea marshes with its clouds of little mauve flowers makes a pretty addition to potpourri or dried flower arrangements.

SOUTHERNWOOD
(Artemisia abrotanum)
Common Names: Lad's Love, Old Man
This low-growing evergreen with small, yellow blossoms and redolent, feathery leaves is a primary ingredient of many potpourris and old-fashioned nosegays. However, the odor of the burning leaves of this herb is pungent. Add it to incense to clear tension and unhappiness from the home, enhance your meditational skills, and destroy cooking and tobacco odors.

SPEARMINT
(Mentha spicata)
This is a Voodoo protection oil for the physical body and home. Add several drops to basil, rosemary, rue, mistletoe, mandrake, and vervain to ward off intruders. A landlord who wants to keep his property rented should mix spearmint, sandalwood powder, and House Blessing powder, and burn it in the apartment. As other mints, spearmint makes an interesting potpourri ingredient. The scent is herbaceous, mellow, and green. The Romans made crowns from spearmint, and it was a favorite Medieval strewing herb.

SPIKENARD
(Nardostachys jatamansi)
This herbaceous plant native to the Himalayas is believed to be the origin of the perfume so cherished by the ancient Egyptians, Sumerians, Hebrews, and Greeks. Since nowadays it is difficult to find the essential oil, many perfumiers substitute lemongrass or lemon verbena for formulas calling for spikenard. The scent is in the roots. It is a shame that spikenard is so hard to come by these days because it makes a perfect fragrance for the New Age, for it

is alleged to expand the consciousness. *Vagnera amplexicaulis* is a wild spikenard with soft-scented, creamy white blossoms that grows in damp American woods.

SPRUCE
(Picea mariana)

The odor of this conifer is lighter than pine or fir, so it makes a fine blender in woodsy, spicy, or flowery perfumes that will not overpower anything. It is a perfect fragrance to inhale in a diffuser when meditating, as it opens the mind to the sephira of Yesod, yet keeps you alert and grounded.

STORAX
(Stryax officinalis, Liquidambar orientalis)
Common Names: Stryax, Sweet Gum

This Mercurian gum fixative hails from Asia Minor, China, and North America. It is the liquid balsam produced from wounds made in a small tree. The resultant amber-colored gum or balsam is collected by Nomads and used commercially as a flavoring, expectorant, and antiseptic. The June-blooming blossoms are also quite fragrant. The fragrance adds a low, dark note to perfume blends.

Storax makes a fine altar incense and is used by the Roman Catholic Church. The aroma, allied to that of benzoin, is like jonquil when distilled. In the Qabala, the scent is associated with the 12th path and also with the tarot trump the Hierophant.

STRAWBERRY
(Fragraria genus)

Fairies are said to love an offering of strawberry oil. The ambrosial scent draws good fortune if added to incense or the bath.

The leaves are a symbol of foresight. Their beauty has inspired emblems for crests of the British gentry as well as crystal patterns. The plump, red fruit inspired its name, "perfect excellence" in the language of flowers. Strawberry and other fruity fragrances are often preferred by children and teens in perfumes, potpourris and cosmetics.

SWEET PEA
(Lathyrus odoratus)

The leaves of this whitish, pinkish, mauve to salmon-colored climbing flower have an exquisite butterfly-like shape resembling cut crystal. The plant was discovered in Sicily, but has been naturalized around the world. The flower's striking beauty has been copied on emblems and coronets of princes, dukes, earls, and marquises.

Some people complain that the sweet pea lately has been cultivated for its lovely blooms rather than the scent, but the *grandifolia* varieties are said to retain a very sweet, soft-hued scent. Some of the more fragrant types were developed by Atlee Burpee, and still can be bought through the company's catalogue.

Sweet pea is alleged to enhance one's attractiveness to strangers, and brings love and loyalty if worn daily. Anoint love sigils with the oil.

SULPHUR

This pale, yellow substance emits an acrid, bitter odor when burned. Use it in banishing, hex removal, and Countermagic incenses. Be sure no animals or children are in the house when you burn sulphur unless you leave the windows open, or they may suffocate.

SWEET FERN
(Comptonia asplenifolia)
Common Name: Sweet Gale

A weedy, wild botanical found along roadsides, the entire plant exudes a spicy, resinous fragrance. It was once believed to cure St. Vitus dance.

TANGERINE
(Citrus nobilis var. *deliciosa)*
Common Name: Mandarin Oil

This spicy citrus fragrance cold pressed from the outer skin of the fruit is said to add zest to rituals and life. It is an ingredient of sexually potent Ishtar massage oil, and lends an exotic note to potpourris and sachets. The scent combines well with coriander, tonka, bergamot, and sandalwood.

TANSY
(Tanacetum vulgare)
Common Name: Golden Buttons

A pungent herb with a tight-headed yellow flower, poisonous to ingest, nonetheless, is useful in potpourris, everlasting arrangements, moth and fly repellents, and closet and drawer refresheners. The longlasting buds do not wither, and the dried botanical lends an herby, but sweet odor to incense. The flower, representing "immortality" in the language of flowers, is one of the "bitter herbs" mentioned in the Bible that the Jews eat at Passover.

THUJA
(Thuja occidentalis)
Common Name: American Arbor Vitae

This conifer, indigenous to North America and China, has an invigorating, piney scent. The essence distilled from the leaves or bark is applied externally for various malignant conditions, cystitis, and warts. Do not ingest the essence in aromatherapy or herbal medicine unless you are under a certified doctor's care, as it is extremely poisonous. The oil made from the distillation of the small branches can be added safely to perfumes and potpourris. The leaves smell like resinous wild strawberries.

THYME
(Thymus vulgaris)

Many varieties of thyme exist, most of them are short, creeping plants. Some smell like camphor, caraway, or lemon, and still others like pineapple. In general, thyme is scented similarly to rosemary, and has the same attributes that improve concentration and memory.

The aroma of this herb when burned is surprisingly delicious. It is an ingredient of home protection incense to keep family members healthy and happy. Thyme is one of the old English herbs used in incenses to enable one to see fairies. It also is an ingredient of Holy Water. Inhale oil of thyme in a steam facial to ease the symptoms of sinusitis and the flu. At the Pasteur Institute in Paris the micro-organism that causes yellow fever was destroyed with thyme, angelica, cinnamon, and sandalwood.

The scent was so revered by the ancients that they claimed their famous writers and sages exuded the smell. The fragrance also lends a woodsy, herby aroma to potpourris and sachets.

In the language of flowers, thyme is equated with "activity." The Greeks thought that it restored their energy. Medieval ladies used to embroider knights' scarves with the image of thyme and a bee.

TOBACCO
(Nicotiana genus)
Many types of tobacco are blended into Shaman, Voodoo, and Macumba incenses to call upon the gods and make them appear before mortals, but the most popular is *N. bigelovii*, known as Indian tobacco. The aroma is said to create an atmosphere conducive to trancework.

TONKA BEAN
(Coumarouma odorata, Dipteryx odorata)
Common Name: Tonquin Bean
Crush or cut the poisonous seeds, and add them to Damballah incense to produce a vanilla-like scent. Pulverized tonka beans can be added to mothproofing sachets. Coumarin, which is the volatile oil of the tonka, is a fixative in potpourri. Magically, apply the scent in healing rituals or in spells to attract fast luck.

TUBEROSE
(Polianthes tuberosa)
The oil, obtained by enfleurage from the waxy, white, tubular-shaped, flowers of this East Indian climbing wild flower, is allegedly worn by men to seduce virtuous ladies. The exotic fragrance fell into disfavor when the flower was brought too much to funerals. Perhaps this is why besides being a love oil the scent is alleged to drive away evil.

In the language of flowers, tuberose means "dangerous pleasures" and "voluptuousness." If a lover receives one of these showy flowers from the hand of his lady, it means "mutual affection."

UVA-URSI
(Arctostaphylos uva-ursi)
Common Names: Kinnikinnick, Bearberry

This is an ingredient of Shaman Vision and other psychic incenses and woodsy blends. The flat, green leaves look pretty in woodsy or herby potpourris. Added to douche water it is said to help alleviate various female complaints.

VALERIAN
(Valeriana officinalis)
Common Names: Garden Heliotrope, Vandalroot, Allheal

Valerian has a strange odor. The flowers smell almost like heliotrope when whiffed from afar, but up close turn fetid. The dried root smells even more obnoxious, but if used parsimoniously in incense, can lend an interestingly tart flavor. Try including some mace to offset the odor. Cats (if you have ever whiffed the canned cat food they go for so much, you won't be surprised) are enamored of the root. Some sweet varieties of valerian exist, including V. celtica, V. elongata, and V. supina. Valerian is an important ingredient of Virgo and Thoth incenses.

VANILLA
(Vanilla planiflora, V. tahitensis)
The pod of a Mexican creeping, greenish-yellow orchid flavors baked goods and sweetens potpourris, perfumes, sachets, and Voodoo love oils. It is said to alleviate frustrations. The tenacious essence attracts peace and love to the home when added to floor wash or sachet. It is alleged to stimulate the mind and promote endurance, inspiration, intuition, patience, and facilitate better organizational skills.

One substitute for vanilla is vanilla-leaf (Achlys triphylla), a coastal plant, the leaves of which strike a delicious note in incenses and potpourris. The terrestial vanilla orchid (Nigritella angustifolia) also may be substituted. This orchid is found in the mountains and pastures of Europe and Siberia. A synthetic vanilla has been synthesized from coal tar!

VERBENA
(Lippia citriodora, Verbena triphylla, Aloysia triphylla)
Common Names: Lemon Verbena, Van-Van

The essence is found in the leaves and stems of the plant. The scent stimulates the brain and improves memory, so may be tried in postoperative cerebral aneurism situations. Verbena also lessens nausea and dizziness. The fragrance combines well with neroli, myrtle, and jasmine. A good substitute for this scent in perfumery is otto of lemongrass.

In ancient Britain, Druidic women wore garlands of verbena like crowns. Anoint mojo bags, roots, and talismans to stimulate creativity. The lemony scent is said to be adored by lovers of the good life. Use the leaves to scent finger bowls. Verbena attracts success to all enterprises and guards against Black Magic. During the sixteenth century mothers anointed their children with the oil because they believed it helped make them quicker at learning and gave them a joyous childhood. In Gem Magic, this scent is associated with chrysolite.

VERVAIN
(Verbena hastata)
Common Name: Blue Vervain

Vervain is an herb employed in small amounts in incense and for protection. The Druids considered this herb sacred and used it together with mistletoe and mandrake to throw curses back on enemies. The Greeks burned it in their auguries to induce a favorable prophecy. In the language of flowers, vervain understandably means "enchantment."

VETIVERT
(Vetivera zizanioides)
Common Name: Khus-Khus

The reddish-brown oil of this tenacious grass grown in India, Burma, Java, Sri Lanka, Kenya, and Central America drives away evil when added to Dragonbane incense. In Victorian times it was used to scent muslin and was a popular fixative in perfumes, smelling somewhat like a dry, woodsy, musty version of violets. As opposed to sandalwood, it is more musty than spicy.

During hot spells in India people would wet down their vetivert-thatched roofs so that as the grass dried it released its cooling fragrance. Vetivert was a primary ingredient of the famous *Bouquet du Roi*, and is also an excellent moth proofer when used as a sachet. In aromatherapy, vetivert cures extreme nervous exhaustion and anorexia. It combines well with rose, cardamom, tonka, neroli, and ylang-ylang.

VIOLET
(Viola odorata)

The smell of violets hidden in the green
Pour'd back into my empty soul and frame
The times when I remember to have been
joyful and free from blame   - Lord Tennyson.

A delightful Greek legend claims that when Zeus changed Io into a white heifer he created white violets in the fields for her to eat. Then Venus, jealous of Cupid's affection for these flowers, turned them all purple. Violets were so cherished that Athenians adopted the flower as the symbol of their city state.

This dainty perfume was popular in Victorian times, and was Empress Josephine's and Elizabeth I's favorite. The fragrance evokes orris root. Of the violet Mohammed is said to have sagely remarked that its scent recalls an atmosphere of warmth in winter and coolness in summer.

Mistakenly it is considered a fragile scent that fades quickly; actually the flower exudes an inhibitor to the sense of smell that makes the scent only seem to fade. It would seem it is impossible to overindulge in this fragrance!

Violet blends well in potpourris and perfumes, and in fact, was the chief flower in perfumery and cooking during the Renaissance. The shy blooms are used as garnishes and ingredients of soups, salads, wines, liqueurs, desserts, and cosmetics.

The scent is said to be worn by the sympathetic and refined. Violets are known to aromatherapists for their expectorant properties. They also are applied in poultices to treat sores, wounds and skin cancer.

The green-colored essence is alleged to break down the barriers of indifference between people and calm strife. The fragrance comforts those whose children have died. For all these reasons violet scent is sometimes called "wings of healing." In the language of flowers violets mean "I am faithful" and "modesty."

WILLOW
(Salix genus)

Bits of the bark of the fragrant *S. balsamifera* are used in lunar incenses. Burning the bark is alleged to promote fertility. In times gone by, peasants sewed willow bark into amulets to protect and bring them good fortune.

WINTERGREEN
(Gaultheria procumbens)
(The *Pyrola* genus is known as Shinleaf.)

Wintergreen combats coughs and bronchitis with its aspirin-like properties, and prevents bladder infections. It lends a strikingly minty note to potpourris with undertones of sassafras, clove, and spice. Most of the wintergreen available for perfumery is synthetic.

WISTERIA
(Wistaria frutescens)
American Wisteria
(W. sinensis alba)

This honey-scented fragrance which comes from the pea-shaped flowers of a climbing vine according to occult perfumery sharpens the intellect and senses, promotes psychic visions, and improves clairvoyant skills. Witches believe that wisteria is the key that unlocks the door to the spirit world. It makes a consummate personal anointing oil.

WOODRUFF
(Asperula odorata)

The plant is also known as sweet woodruff because of the delightful vanilla-like scent emitted by the burning leaves. It is also a classic ingredient in potpourri and sachet.

YERBA SANTA
(Eriodictyon californicum)

Also known as holy herb, this native of Southern California is used medicinally by the Indians. The leaves emit a strong fragrance when crushed.

YLANG-YLANG
(Cananga odorata)

The name means "flower of flowers," which is quite approprite, since the essence steam distilled from the greenish-yellowish-white bell-shaped, drooping flowers of a tall Malaysian evergreen tree is redolent of hyacinth, jasmine, lilac, narcisssus, and clove, and blends well with these scents. The essence is hypotensive and antiseptic.

Wear this provocatively, sexual scent when you want to surprise your lover with a divine night of love. Add sparingly to blends that include neroli, jasmine, and sandalwood, as the scent is sticky and sweet, and can be overpowering. In aromatherapy, the flower lowers blood pressure, relaxes the facial muscles, and is good for PMS and depression. The fragrance is associated with the watermelon tourmaline in Gem Magic.

Appendix II

Miscellaneous Formulas
for Occult Perfume Oils

These perfumes are measured by parts; for example, 2 = 2 parts of the whole. (d) = drop; 3 d. = 3 drops. The formulas are based on quantities for 1 dram or 1/4 ounce bottles.

The Planets

Sun: 2 frankincense, 1/2 bayberry, 3 d. almond, 1/2 cinnamon, 1 peony, 1 d. chamomile.

Moon: 1 jasmine, 1 lotus, 1/2 magnolia, 1/4 mimosa, 1/4 copaiba, 1/4 honey.

Mars: 2 scotch broom, 1 honeysuckle, 1 dragon's blood (equal parts amber, jasmine, rose, musk).

Mercury: 2 sandalwood, 1/4 cinnamon, 3 d. lavender, 1/2 neroli, 1 muguet.

Jupiter: 1/2 myrrh, 1 jasmine, 1/2 carnation, 6 d. clove, 1/4 oakmoss, 1/4 clover, 1/4 nutmeg.

Venus: 2 sandalwood, 1 white rose, 1/2 violet.

Saturn: 1 myrrh, 6 d. juniper, 2 dark musk, 1/2 cypress.

Neptune: 1 amber, 2 lotus, 1/2 oakmoss, 1 dark musk, 1/4 fern, 1 syringa.

Uranus: 1 hyacinth, 1/2 lily, 1/2 ambergris, 1/2 fir.

Pluto: 1/2 ambergris, 2 stephanotis, 1/4 opoponax, 1/2 datura, 3 d. labdanum.

The Zodiac

Aries: 1 myrrh, 5 d. rosemary, 1/2 geranium rose, 1/2 pine, 1/2 ylang-ylang, 1/4 copaiba.

Taurus: 1/2 red rose, 1 muguet, 1/4 oakmoss, 1/2 frankincense, 1 tuberose.

Gemini: 1/2 rose, 1 lily-of-the-valley, 3 d. lavender, 2 sandalwood, 1/4 civet 1/2 lilac.

Cancer: 2 honeysuckle, 1 jasmine, 1/2 light musk, 6 d. lotus.

Leo: 1 frankincense, 3 d cinnamon, 5 d. pineapple, 1 heliotrope, 1/4 spruce.

Virgo: 1 narcissus, 1/4 hyacinth, 1/2 muguet, 2 sandalwood, 1/2 heliotrope.

Libra: 1 sandalwood, 2 rose, 1/4 violet, 3 d. cherry, 1/2 light musk, 1/2 tuberose.

Scorpio: 2 heather, 1 dark musk, 1/2 myrrh or civet.

Sagittarius: 6 d. spruce, 1 frankincense, 1 myrrh, 1/4 cinnamon, 1 Oriental musk.

Capricorn: 1 myrrh, 1 dark musk, 1/2 lily-of-the-valley, 6 d. patchouly.

Aquarius: 1 frankincense, 1 wild rose, 6 d. coconut, 1/2 cypress, 1/4 ambergris, 1/2 honeysuckle.

Pisces: 2 amber, 1 myrrh, 1 d. mint, 1 lily.

Endnotes

1. *The Bible*, Exodus, Chapter 30, Verse 34.

2. Richard Miller and Iona Miller, *Magical and Ritual Use of Perfumes*, Rochester, Vermont, Destiny Books, 1990, p. 19.

3. Morwyn, *Web of Light: Rites for Witches in the New Age*, Atglen, Pennsylvania, Whitford Press, 1993, pp. 17-18.

4. Gareth Knight, *A Practical Guide to Qabalistic Symbolism: On the Spheres of the Tree of Life*, vol. I, Great Britain, Helios Book Service, 1976 rpt. 1965, pp. 138-144.

5. Morwyn, *Secrets of a Witch's Coven*, West Chester, Pennsylvania, Whitford Press, 1988, pp. 100-103.

6. Louise M. Gruenberg, *Potpourri: The Art of Fragrance Crafting*, Norway, Iowa, Frontier Cooperative Herbs, 1990 rpt. 1984, pp. 80-81.

7. Lady Sara Cunningham-Carter, *The Book of Light*, New York, Magickal Childe Publishing, Inc., 1974, p. 98.

8. Mary Chamberlain, *Old Wives Tales*, London, Virago, 1981, p. 146.

9. Jean Valnet, *The Practice of Aromatherapy: Holistic Health and the Essential Oils of Flowers and Herbs*, New York, Destiny Books, 1982 p. 26.

10. Sharon Begley and Elizabeth Jones, "Research Amid the Camellias," *Newsweek*, May 15, 1989.

11. Stephen Foster, "Garden Pharmacy," *Harrowsmith*, November/December, 1988.

12. Franz Bardon, *The Practice of Magical Evocation*, Wuppertal, Germany, Dieter Ruggeberg, 1975, p. 164.

13. C.W. Septimus Piesse, *The Art of Perfumery*, Philadelphia, Lindsay and Blakiston, 1867, p. 84.

14. C.A. Nagle, *Magical Charms, Potions and Secrets for Love*, Minneapolis, Minnesota, Marlar Publishing Co., 1972, p. 7.

15. Henri Gamache, *The Magic of Herbs*, Highland Falls, New York, Sheldon Publications, 1942, p. 42.

16. *The Art of Perfumery*, p. 102.

17. *The Practice of Aromatherapy*, pp. 141-142.

18. Susanne Fischer-Rizzi, *Complete Aromatherapy Handbook: Essential Oils for Radiant Health*, New York, Sterling Publishing Co., Inc., 1990, p. 114.

19. In Louise Beebe Wilder, *The Fragrant Garden*. New York: Dover Publications, Inc., 1974 rpt. 1932, pp. 290-291.

20, Wilder, p. 103.

21. *Complete Aromatherapy Handbook*, p. 138.

22. In Eleanour Sinclair Rohde, *A Garden of Herbs*, New York, Dover Publications, Inc., 1969 rpt. 1936, p. 251.

23. *The Fragrant Garden*, p. 68.

24. Anna Riva, *The Modern Herbal Spellbook*, Toluca Lake, California, International Imports, 1974, p. 47.

25. *The Art of Perfumery*, p. 147.

26. Mellie Uyldert, *The Psychic Garden: Plants and Their Esoteric Relationship with Man*, Great Britain, Thorsons Publishers, Ltd., 1980, p. 120.

Bibliography

Books

Aima, *Ritual Book of Herbal Spells*. U.S.A.: Foibles Publications, 1980 rpt. 1976.

Anon. *The Ancient Book of Formulas*. Dallas, Texas: Dorene Publishing Co., Inc., 1967.

Bardon, Franz, *The Practice of Magical Evocation: Instructions for Invoking Spirits from the Spheres Surrounding Us*. Wuppertal, Germany: Dieter Ruggeberg, 1975.

Bayard, Tania. *Sweet Herbs and Sundry Flowers: Medieval Gardens and Gardens of the Cloisters*. New York: The Metropolitan Museum of Art, 1985.

Bethel, May. *The Healing Power of Herbs*. London: Thorsons, 1968.

Chamberlain, Mary. *Old Wives' Tales: Their History, Remedies and Spells*. Great Britain: Virago Press, 1981.

Claremont, Lewis de. *Legends of Incense Herb and Oil Magic*. Revised Edition. Dallas, Texas: Dorene Publishing Co., Inc., 1966 rpt. 1938.

Conway, David. *Ritual Magic: An Occult Primer.* New York: E.P. Dutton, 1978 rpt. 1972.

Culpeper, Nicolas. *Culpeper's Complete Herbal.* New York: W. Foulsham and Company, Ltd., nd.

Cunningham-Carter, Lady Sara. *A Witch's Herbal.* unpublished ms.

———. *The Book of Light.* New York: Magickal Childe Publishing, Inc., 1974.

Donahue, Carloetta. *The Older Skin.* West Palm Beach, Florida: Globe Mini Mag, nd.

Editors. *Magic and Medicine of Plants.* Pleasantville, New York: The Reader's Digest Association, Inc., 1986.

Fettner, Ann Tucker. *Potpourri, Incense and Other Fragrant Concoctions.* New York: Workmen Publishing Co., 1977 rpt 1972.

Fischer-Rizzi, Susanne. *Complete Aromatherapy Handbook: Essential Oils for Radiant Health.* New York: Sterling Publishing Company, Inc., 1990. Translated from the German by Elisabeth E. Reinersmann.

Foley, Daniel J., ed. *Herbs for Use and Delight: An Anthology from the Herbarist.* New York: Dover Publications, Inc., 1974.

Frazier, Gregory and Beverly. *The Bath Book.* San Francisco: Troubador Press, 1973.

Gamache, Henri. *The Magic of Herbs.* Highland Falls, New York: Sheldon Publishing, 1942.

Green, Marian. *The Elements of Natural Magic.* Great Britain: Element Books, n.d.

Grieve, Mrs. M. *A Modern Herbal.* 2 vols. New York: Dover Publications, Inc., 1971, rpt. 1931.

Gruenberg, Louise M. and Ronda L. Brets, Contributing Author. *Potpourri: The Art of Fragrance Crafting.* Norway, Iowa: Frontier Cooperative Herbs, 1990, rpt. 1987.

Howard, Michael. *Incense and Candle Burning: The Practice and Purpose of a Simple Magical Art.* New, expanded and revised edition. Great Britain: The Aquarian Press, 1991.

Jangl, Alda Marian and James Francis Jangl. *Ancient Legends of the Twelve Birthflowers.* Coeur D'Alene, Idaho: Prisma Press, 1986.

Keller, Mitzie Stuart. *Mysterious Herbs and Roots: Ancient Secrets for Beautie, Health, Magick, Prevention and Youth.* Culver City, California: Peace Press, Inc., 1978.

Knight, Gareth. *A Practical Guide to Qabalistic Symbolism.* 2 vols. Great Britain: Helios Book Service Publications, Ltd., 1976 rpt. 1965.

Lavabre, Marcel F. *Aromatherapy Workbook.* Rochester, Vermont: Healing Arts Press, 1990.

Manniche, Lise. *An Ancient Egyptian Herbal.* London: British Museum Press, 1993 rpt. 1989.

Maury, Marguerite. *Marguerite Maury's Guide to Aromatherapy: The Secrests of Life and Youth: a Modern Alchelmy.* English Translation. Great Britain: Danielle Ryman, 1989.

Miller, Alan Richard and Iona Miller. *The Magical and Ritual Use of Perfumes.* Rochester, Vermont: Destiny Books, 1990.

Nagle, C.A. *Magical Charms, Potions and Secrets for Love.* Minneapolis, Minnesota: Marlar Publishing Co, 1972.

Naves, J. R. and G. Mazuyer. *Natural Perfume Materials: A Study of Concretes, Resinoids, Floral Oils and Pomades.* New York: Reinhold Publishing Corporation, 1947.

Pickston, Margaret. *The Language of Flowers.* Great Britain: Michael Joseph Ltd., 1973 rpt. 1968.

Piesse, G. W. Septimus. *The Art of Perfumery, and the Methods of Obtaining the Odors of Plants.* Philadelphia: Lindsay and Blakiston, 1867.

Powell, Claire. *The Meaning of Flowers: A Garland of Plant Lore and Symbolism from Popular Customs and Literature.* Boulder, Colorado: Shambhala Publications, Inc., 1979.

Riva, Anna. *Magic with Incenses and Powders.* Toluca Lake, California: International Imports, 1988.

———. *Golden Secrets of Mystic Oils.* Toluca Lake, California: International Imports, 1978.

———. *The Modern Herbal Spellbook.* Toluca Lake, California: International Imports, 1974.

Rohde, Eleanour Sinclair. *A Garden of Herbs.* Revised and Enlarged Edition. New York: Dover Publications, Inc., 1969 rpt. 1936.

Rose, Jeanne. *Herbs and Things: Jeanne Rose's Herbal.* New York: Workmen Publishing Co., 1977 (rpt 1972).

———. *Jeanne Rose's Kitchen Cosmetics: Choosing and Using Countryside Ingredients to Make Natural Concoctions.* New York and Wellingborough, England: Thorsons Publishing Group, 1978.

Schoen, Linda Allen, ed. *The AMA Book of Skin and Hair Care.* Philadelphia and New York: J.B. Lippincott Co., 1976 (rpt 1971).

Smith, Steven R. *Wylundt's Book of Incense*. York Beach, Maine: Samuel Weiser, Inc., 1992.

Tisserand, Robert B. *The Art of Aromatherapy: The Healing and Beautifying Properties of the Essential Oils of Flowers and Herbs*. New York: Destiny Books, 1983 rpt 1977.

Trueman, John. *The Romantic Story of Scent*. Great Britain: Aldus Books Ltd., 1975.

Uyldert, Mellie. *The Psychic Garden: Plants and Their Esoteric Relationship with Man*. Trans. from Dutch by H.A. Smith. Great Britain: Thorsons Publishers, Ltd, 1980.

Valnet, Jean. *The Practice of Aromatherapy: Holistic Health and the Essential Oils of Flowers and Herbs*. New York: Destiny Books, 1982. English translation copyrighted by The C.W. Daniel Company Ltd., 1982.

Vinci, Leo. *Incense: Its Ritual Significance, Use and Preparation*. New York: Samuel Weiser, Inc., 1980.

Wakefield, Grace M. *Decorating with Fragrance: The Potpourri Story*. Chincoteague, Virginia: Tom Thumb Workshops, 1981.

Walker, Elizabeth. *Making Things with Herbs*. New Canaan, Connecticut: Kent Publishing Co., 1977.

Wilder, Louise Beebe. *The Fragrant Garden A Book About Sweet Scented Flowers and Leaves*. New York: Dover Publications, Inc., 1974, rpt. 1932.

Articles

Begley, Sharon and Elizabeth Jones. "Research Amid the Camellias." *Newsweek*, May 15, 1989.

———. "Zombies and Other Mysteries: Ethnobotanists Seek Magical, Medicinal Plants." *Newsweek*, February 22, 1988.

Brody, Jane E."How We Smell May Lead to Better Health." *The New York Times*, Tuesday, February 23, 1993.

Danbom, Dan. "Smell of Success." *Registered Representative*. May, 1991.

Darnton, Nina. "The Politics of Bath Oil: A Whiff of Concern." *Newsweek*, October 21, 1990.

Foster, Stephen. "Garden Pharmacy." *Harrowsmith*, November/ December, 1988.

Glick, Daniel. "New Age Meets Hippocrates: Medicine Gets Serious About Unconventional Therapy." *Newsweek*, July 13, 1992.

Krantz, Michael. "Two Scents Worth: A New Fragrance Company Takes Advantage of Pheromones." *Omni*, January, 1994.

Lewis, Stephanie. "Aromas That Are Heaven Scent." *The London Times*, Weekend, Saturday, April 9, 1994.

Mason, Diane. "Making Scents of It All." *The St. Petersburg Times*, Friday, June 7, 1991.

Meyer, Scott. "Create Your Own Botanical Bodycare." *Organic Gardening*, December, 1991.

O'Neill, Molly. "Taming the Frontier of the Senses: Using Aromas to Manipulate Moods." *The New York Times*, Wednesday, November 27, 1991.

Pleasant, Barbara. "Edible Bouquet." *Organic Gardening*, January, 1989.

Ruben, Rik. "Nosing Around: Studies Discover Smell Can Affect Work Performance." *Boulder Daily Camera*, Thursday, May 30, 1991, rpt. from *Dallas Morning News*.